Providing Emergency Care

David F. Foulk, Ed. D.
Georgia Southern College
and
Mark B. Dignan, Ph. D.
*The Bowman Gray School of Medicine
of Wake Forest University*

Hunter Textbooks Inc.

SPECIAL ACKNOWLEDGMENTS

Cover photograph copyright 1988 by Tyler Cox.   Models (left to right): Danny and Amy Crouse; and Ellen Severt

Text illustrations (unless otherwise noted) by Robin Rice, copyright 1989 by Hunter Textbooks Inc.

Illustrations in Chapter 3 are reproduced with permission of the American Heart Association, copyright JAMA, June 6, 1986, American Heart Association.

CPR/ECC Performance Sheets appearing at the end of Chapter 3 are reproduced with permission of the American Heart Association, copyright CPR/ECC Performance Sheets, American Heart Association.

The following manufacturers have granted permission to use illustrations of their equipment and supplies:
Hare traction splint by DYNA MED, Carlsbad, CA
Sager emergency traction splint, Minto Research, Redding, CA
E-Collar, Medical Specialties, Charlotte, NC
Stiffneck Cervical Collar, California Medical Products, Long Beach, CA
Philadelphia Cervical Collar, Philadelphia Cervical Co., Westville, NJ
AnaKit, Miles Laboratories AiInc., West Haven, CT
Johnson and Johnson, New Brunswick, NJ

Inquiries should be addressed to:

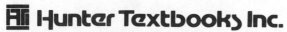 **Hunter Textbooks Inc.**

823 Reynolda Road
Winston-Salem, North Carolina 27104

Preface

This book was developed to as a practical guide for providing emergency care to those with sudden illness and injuries. The emphasis is on thoughtful, careful assessment of the victim, understanding common injuries and illnesses, and provision of basic emergency care. We believe that this book can be used for basic training for professionals as well as for training interested lay persons.

The need for emergency care is a constant in our complex society. In spite of our best efforts, accidents happen and people are injured. Sudden illness may also develop without warning, away from medical care. It is interesting to note that even with the tremendous advances in our ability to effectively treat the injured, the initial emergency care given remains one of the most important predictors of the outcome for the victim. Because doctors, nurses and other highly trained emergency care professionals cannot be everywhere, lay people are often the first called upon to give emergency care. With these considerations in mind, we have produced a text that is oriented toward practical application of principles of emergency care. Our goal in writing this text has been to emphasize basic principles of emergency care that preserve life and prevent further injury. Because it is the most basic principle of emergency care, an entire chapter is devoted to *asessment* of the victim. All chapters that follow reinforce the importance of assessment.

The organization of this book is around sound principles of emergency care. The first three chapters focus on fundamentals: Basic principles of emergency care, assessment of the victim, and restoring respiration and heartbeat. The skills included in these chapters are critical to preserving life in an emergency situation. Basic anatomy and physiology are presented in the first chapter and reintroduced as needed in the text. Because injuries usually involve multiple body systems, presentation of emergency care is organized around injury type and not body system. Emphasis is on integrating relevant anatomy and physiology with assessment and emergency care. Injuries to specific body systems such as the central nervous system are presented as relevant to discussion of specific emergency care situations. Additionally, because of the increased risks faced by emergency caregivers, we have carefully woven in, throughout the text, practical precautions and recommendations for preventing accidental infection with communicable diseases such as hepatitis and AIDS .

Wounds, bleeding control and shock are covered in the fourth chapter, followed by bone and joint injuries in the fifth. The sixth chapter discusses moving the injured while preventing further injuries. These chapters emphasize developing an understanding of injuries coupled with a complete, practical explanation of how to provide proper emergency care. Burns, heat exhaustion, heat stroke, frostbite and hypothermia are the topics included in the chapter that follows. Proper emergency care of victims with these conditions requires careful training in conducting a thorough assessment followed by quick action.

The final chapters of the text include discussions of poisoning, medical emergencies, out-of-hospital childbirth and crisis control. Each of these chapters includes discussion on assessment of the victim and techniques for providing emergency care.

Chapter Eleven discusses the social and emotional aspects of accidents and injuries, a subject often overlooked in emergency care training. Injured or severely ill people are often traumatized by their experience, and the emergency caregiver should be equipped to recognize signs of uncontrolled emotional distress and provide care. Effective emergency care for emotional distress requires reaching out to the victim with compassion and empathy. This chapter also discusses the emergency care aspects of drug and alcohol abuse, emphasizing dealing effectively with the disturbance of behavior that often accompanies these situations.

Each chapter in this book is accompanied by exercises designed to help the reader apply the information given and practice related skills. Emergency care is skills based, and practice is necessary to achieve competence. Additional emergency care scenarios are provided at the end of the book to help the reader practice incorporating skills as needed to provide care for accident victims.

Acknowledgements

Many people and organizations have helped us in preparing this manuscript. Dr. Jack Ellison at the University of Tennessee was our mentor in teaching emergency care. Dr. Ellison's gift for understanding the need for teaching principles of emergency care in an environment that fosters learning have not been lost on us.

For production of this book we are indebted to Tyler Cox and Dan Crouse for their professionalism in providing many of the photographs needed. Emergency care teaching requires demonstration, and their patience and helpfulness were appreciated. Ernestine Godfrey and her staff at Hunter Textbooks have our gratitude and admiration for their endless patience and good cheer throughout the preparation of this book.

Finally, Counts Rescue Equipment and Mr. Ed Hampton have been very helpful to us in providing access to the many companies producing the newest emergency care products.

Contents

Chapter One
Introduction
Guidelines for Giving Emergency Care

Accidental injuries in the home, automobile accidents, mishaps that occur on the job, and sudden illnesses all have one thing in common. Even though they vary in seriousness, all are situations in which the injured person may need immediate care—care that will stabilize the person and reduce the chance of further injury until professional medical care can be obtained.

Emergency care training is designed to enable you to provide this immediate care. Knowledge and skills in providing emergency care are extremely valuable, because accidents are the leading cause of death and disability among the youngest and oldest age groups in America. Furthermore, in many cases, it is not the accidental injury that is responsible for death or disability, but a lack of competent emergency care at the scene of the accident. In most cases, a skilled caregiver can improve the outcome of an accident by applying first aid procedures at the accident scene that will minimize damage and speed recovery.

BASIC GUIDELINES

Regardless of the nature of the injury, as an emergency caregiver you need to be guided by basic principles or guidelines. These principles are based on common sense combined with extensive experience with traumatic injuries.

Four basic guidelines are essential to first aid. These principles are based on the premise that quick action can preserve life and speed recovery by minimizing damage from injury. In order of importance, these basic guidelines are as follows:

FIRST   **Act to provide an open airway.**

SECOND   **Insure adequate ventilation (breathing).**

THIRD   **Insure circulation (heartbeat).**

FOURTH   **Stop severe bleeding.**

Other injuries may be very serious indeed, but if the victim is not breathing, has no heartbeat, or is bleeding uncontrollably, he or she is not likely to live regardless of other injuries.

Keeping Your Emotions in Check

Situations in which a person has been injured or suddenly taken ill can be emotionally disturbing. Emotional upset often clouds judgment. As a caregiver, it is crucial that you adopt an objective attitude and try to insulate yourself from emotional attachment that will cloud your judgment. Professional action requires a professional attitude. The injured person and bystanders are also calmed by an attitude that is compassionate, but in control emotionally.

Title	Hours of Training	Subject Matter	Audience
First Aider	12-40	Boy and Girl Scouts, American Red Cross, School Programs	Open to the public
First Responder	90	General first aid with special emphasis on awareness of environmental injuries	Those working in hazardous occupations or dangerous environments
Emergency Medical Technician (EMT)	120	First Responder training plus use of oxygen and advanced shock first aid	Open to the public*; regulated by the US Dept. of Transportation (DOT)
Paramedic	200+	Advanced training: Intravenous fluid administration, ECGs, Drug administration, other advanced procedures	Requires EMT training and experience

*Local requirements vary; some communities require previous training and/or minimum educational levels.

RESOURCES

Tremendous strides have been made in providing first aid and emergency care services to the public through the course of the past two decades. One of the most important of these advances has been the development of several levels of training. (See chart above.)

At the level of this text, you will become trained to perform valuable lifesaving procedures as well as to provide first aid for common, everyday injuries. As the level of training increases, the level of emergency care also increases in depth and extent, to the level of providing services that closely parallel those available in the most modern hospital.

As training programs have developed, means for communication among the public, professional emergency caregivers and health care facilities have also improved. In many parts of America, Emergency Medical Systems (EMS) are organized systems that have been established to coordinate services. The familiar 911 telephone system has been extremely useful in eliminating confusion about notifying professionals in emergency situations.

Where EMS systems are not developed, the citizen who needs emergency care is often faced with determining the agency serving his or her geographic area (and even the type of emergency, in some cases) before help can be summoned.

CALLING FOR HELP: DOS AND DON'TS

When an emergency arises and help is needed from the police, a rescue squad, or fire department, clear communication is imperative. Unfortunately, the nature of an emergency situation makes communication more difficult than normal. People are usually upset and in a great hurry—two factors that obviously hinder communication. Here are some simple rules that will insure the need for help is communicated clearly.

1. Tell the operator
   —where the help is needed.
   —the phone number you are using.
   —what happened.
   —how many people need help.
   —what is being done now.

2. In communicating directions to the operator, try to give landmarks to help identify the location. Street addresses may be insufficient.

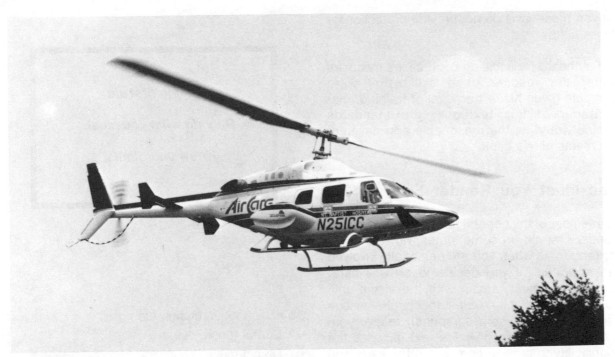

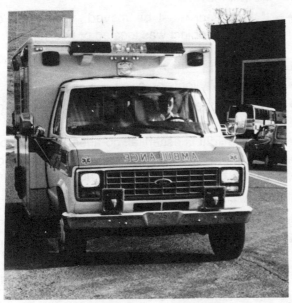

Modern emergency transport resources make getting to the hospital faster and safer than ever. The vital link remains the quality of first aid provided before professional help arrives.

3. **Do not hang up** the telephone until the person on the other end of the phone does so. It is not uncommon for people to call 911 in an emergency and forget to give the address where help is needed. Staying on the line until the other person hangs up will help prevent unclear communication.

4. If possible, station a person by the road to wait for the rescuers. This person will be able to signal the rescuers and save valuable time spent looking for a house number.

EMERGENCY CARE AND THE LAW

Understanding the rights and responsibilities of the injured and those who render aid to them is important. The person who provides emergency care is protected to varying degrees by "Good Samaritan" laws. These laws vary from state to state but, in essence, they protect the rescuer who provides assistance in an unofficial capacity.

However, these laws do not provide protection for reckless behavior.

The standard for deciding court cases has been whether the rescuer used skills that were reasonable given his or her level of training. For the reader of this textbook, the standards expected would be the reasonable application of the contents of this book.

When Must You Render First Aid?

No member of the general public is ever required to render first aid. In some states, however, you must render aid when you are personally involved in an accident. If you decide to provide care, however, you must remain with the victim until rescuers with official medical authority (fire, rescue squad, emergency room personnel) relieve you. Thus, the decision to give first aid includes the responsibility to provide care within the limits and standards of your training as well as the responsibility to continue giving care until you are relieved.

Consent

Everyone has the right to accept or to refuse first aid. In cases where a victim refuses first aid but appears to be injured to the extent that his or her condition will worsen without care, you should stay with the victim. In many cases, the victim will accept care as the seriousness of the injuries becomes clear.

Crime Scenes

When a crime may have been committed and you are giving first aid at the scene, your actions are important to the victim as well as the police. Precautions should be taken to insure that pertinent evidence is not destroyed through carelessness. The following are suggestions for action at a crime scene when you must provide first aid before the police arrive.

Weapons
- Do not touch.
- Do not pick up.
- Note any movement made necessary in giving first aid.

> *In giving first aid:*
>
> *Only do what you must.*
>
> *Know your limits.*

Objects (tables, chairs, etc.)
- Do not touch.
- Do not move.
- If an object must be moved, make note of where the object was located or positioned.

Lighting
- Do not turn lights on or off.
- Do not open or close curtains, shades, or blinds.
- If more light is essential, go ahead and turn on the lights or open the curtains, shades, or blinds, but be sure to inform the police of what you have done.

Washing
- Do not wash yourself in the bathroom, kitchen, or utility room.
- If you must wash yourself, do it outside the area of the crime scene.
- Do not use the garden hose.

Moving the Victim
- If the victim must be moved, note the position of the victim in relation to furniture or other objects.
- Note the condition of the victim's clothing and how it was arranged on the victim.
- Pass this information on to the police.

Deceased Person
- If you touch the person, note where you touched and what you found.

4

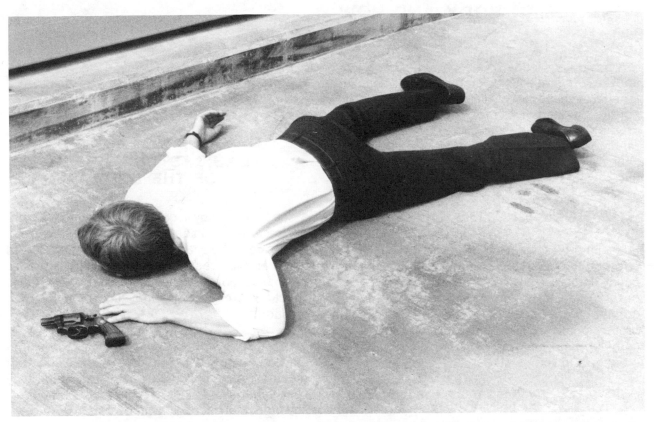

Some situations clearly show foul play. . . or do they? Whether a crime or suicide or accident, the emergency caregiver must approach scenes like this one as though a crime was committed.

Odors

- Note any unusual odors such as drugs, petroleum products, natural gas, alcohol, or other unusual products.
- Inform the police of what you have smelled.

Sightseers

- Keep non-essential personnel away from the scene.

Appliances

- Do not touch air conditioning, appliances, or anything that can be turned on and off.
- If you must touch any control switches, make sure you inform the police of what you did.

Telephone

- If the receiver is off, do not hang it up.
- Do not use the telephone to make calls.
- If communication is necessary, use a neighbor's phone or a public phone.

Covering Deceased Person

- You should not cover a deceased person with a sheet or blanket unless you are instructed to do so by a police officer.
- A sheet or blanket could remove trace evidence such as fingerprints (which can last up to two hours on the deceased person), fibers, and hair.

THE HUMAN BODY AND HOW IT WORKS

A basic knowledge of the parts of the human body and their functions is an essential ingredient for effectiveness in providing emergency care. It is not the purpose of this textbook to teach human anatomy and physiology; however, further readings (a list is included at the end of this chapter) are available to help you learn more about this subject.

THE BODY AND ITS MOVEMENTS

Health professionals use specific terminology to describe the body and its functions. As an emergency caregiver, it is important to have a basic understanding of such language in order to communicate effectively with other health professionals. While thousands of terms are in common use, knowing this simple list will be of great help to you:

Anterior: referring to the front (face side) of the body

Posterior: referring to the back side of the body

Superior: toward the head and away from the feet

Inferior: toward the feet and away from the head

Midline: an imaginary division of the body into right and left halves

Medial: toward the midline

Lateral: away from the midline

Proximal: closer to the midline

Distal: farther away from the midline

Abduction: to move away from the midline

Adduction: to move toward the midline

Flex: to bend at a joint and move the distal part closer to the rest of the body

Extend: to straighten a joint and move the distal part away from the rest of the body

Supine: lying on the back of the body

Prone: lying on the front of the body

BASIC STRUCTURES OF THE BODY

The human body is composed of a large number of structures, all integrated to allow us to function as we do. Clear and consistent descriptions of these structures are essential to effective communication. For ease of discussion, these structures are grouped into categories with similar function.

Topographical Anatomy. The surface of the body can be divided into a large number of regions, each of which can be described by specific terms. Figure 1-1 summarizes the most important of these regions and terms.

Bones and Joints. Since they are often the focus of concern for the emergency caregiver, it is important to know the structure of the arms and legs and their movement. In assessment, lack of motion of a limb or an unexpected position are often the first clues about the nature of an injury. Figures 1-2 and 1-3 summarize the basic skeletal structures of the human body.

Circulation. The cardiovascular system provides for circulation of blood throughout the body. Beginning in the heart and brain (the brain controls the heart), blood that has been used in the tissues returns to the heart and is pumped to the lungs where carbon dioxide and oxygen are exchanged. The freshly-oxygenated blood then returns to the heart and is redistributed to the rest of the body. The major arteries and veins of the body are shown in Figures 1-4 and 1-5.

Nervous System. Sensation of the environment, control of muscles, breathing and heartbeat are all controlled by the brain through the nervous system. The nervous system has many more functions than those mentioned here, of course. Basically, the nervous system provides the "electrical system" for the body.

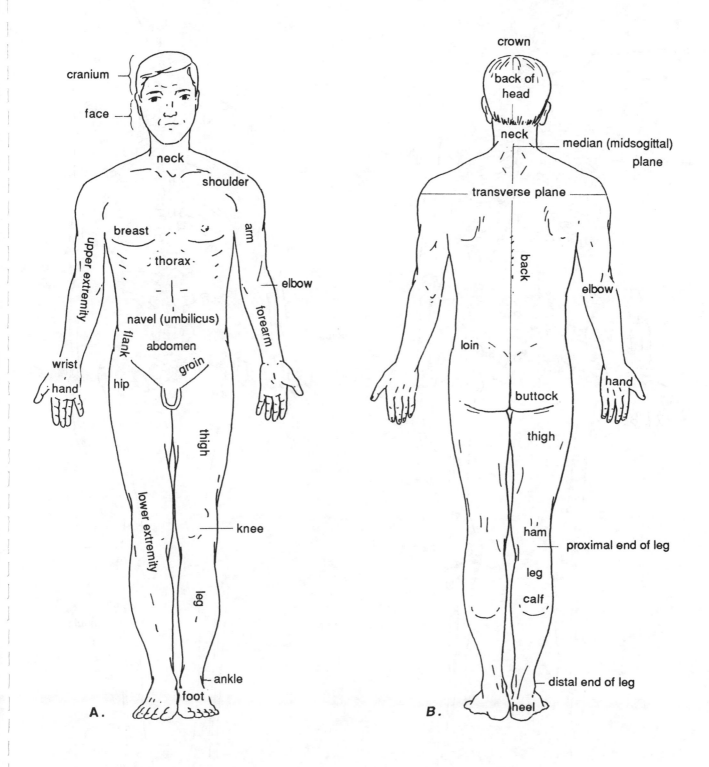

Figure 1-1. *The human figure in anatomical position.*
A, Anterior view; B, Posterior view.

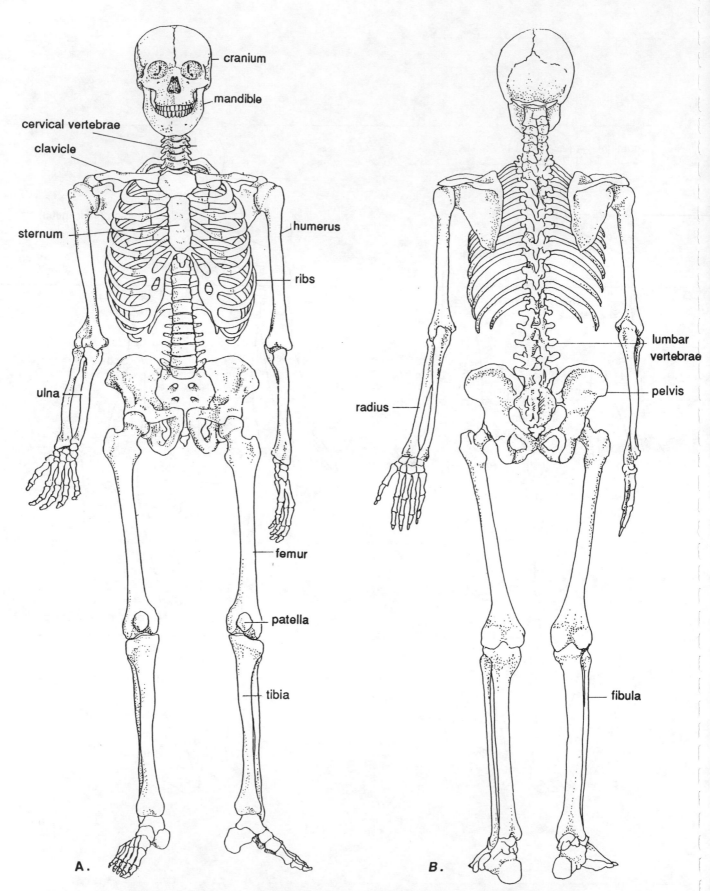

cranium

mandible

cervical vertebrae

clavicle

sternum

humerus

ribs

ulna

lumbar vertebrae

radius

pelvis

femur

patella

tibia

fibula

A.

B.

Figure 1-2. *The human skeleton as projected on the surface of the body.*
A, Anterior view; B, Posterior view.

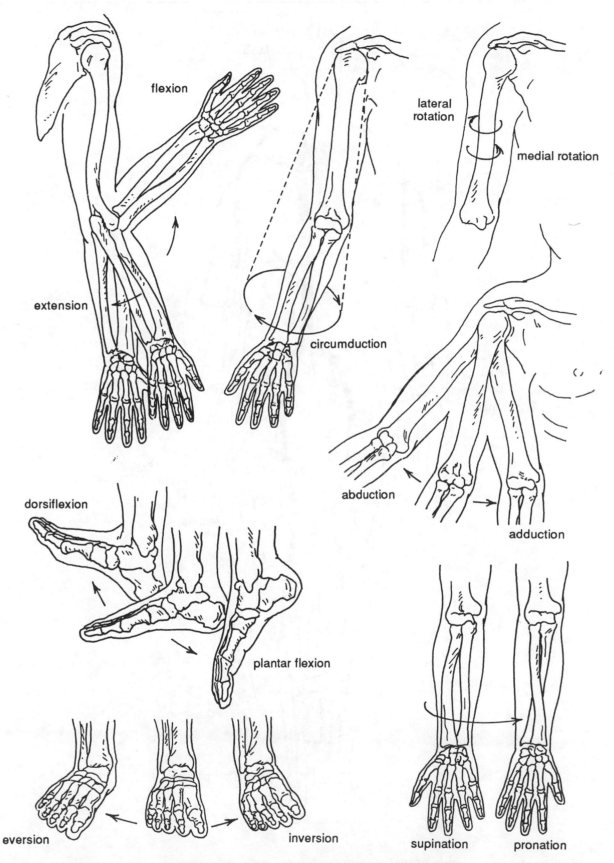

Figure 1-3. *Various movements in articulation.*

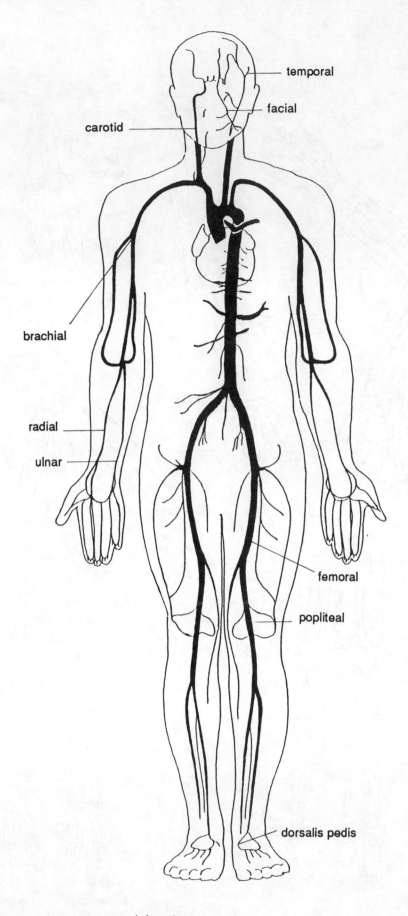

Figure 1-4. *The human arterial system.*

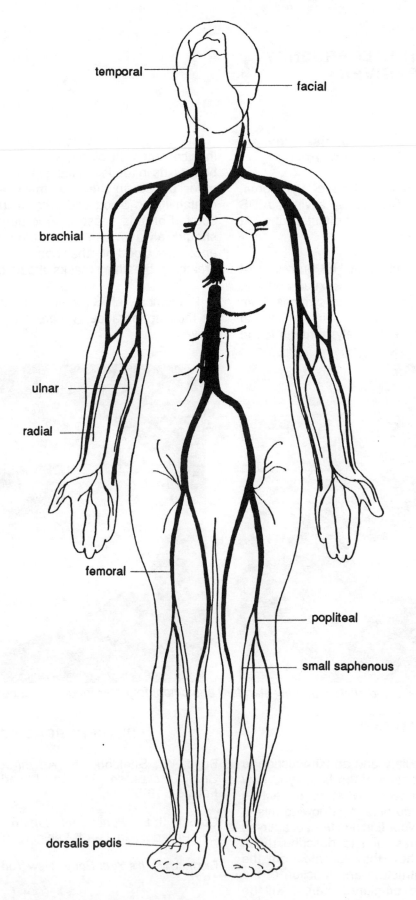

Figure 1-5. *The human venous system.*

AIDS AND THE EMERGENCY CAREGIVER

Protect yourself:

**Where there is blood, use gloves.
Use a mask for rescue breathing.**

AIDS, Acquired Immune Deficiency Syndrome, is a deadly disease. Caused by a virus, AIDS reduces the body's ability to fight off infections. At present, there is no cure.

AIDS is spread through a number of mechanisms, chiefly through sexual contact, through contaminated needles and syringes, from infected mothers to their unborn children during pregnancy or at birth, and (rarely) through blood transfusions.

Emergency caregivers are very likely to come into contact with blood, vomit, saliva and other body fluids in rendering first aid. Scratches, cuts or other breaks in the skin make it possible for contaminated blood and other fluids to enter the body. For this reason, emergency caregivers should always use latex gloves when they encounter blood or other body fluids. For rescue breathing, breathing masks should be used.

Remember, AIDS patients cannot be identified by their appearance. *Where there's blood, use gloves.*

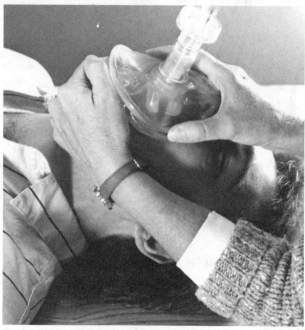 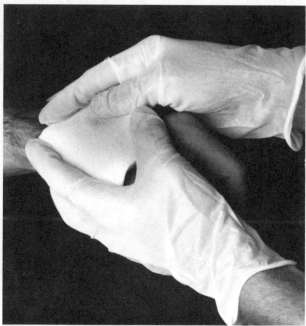

Rescue breathing masks and gloves are now standard equipment for emergency personnel.

SUMMARY

With a basic vocabulary and an introduction to the structures and function of the body, you now have a basis for knowing what to expect in examining the *uninjured* person. Knowing this, it is possible to catalog your findings from examining a person *with* injuries, and to describe these injuries in terms of how they deviate from the normal state. The structure and function of the body, in normal and uninjured states, will be explored in greater detail in upcoming chapters.

FURTHER READINGS

Boyd, W., Sheldon, H. *An Introduction to the Study of Disease.* 7th Ed., Philadelphia, Lea & Febiger, 1977.

Crouch, J. E. *Functional Human Anatomy,* 3rd. Ed. Philadelphia, Lea & Febiger, 1978.

Elson, L.M. *It's Your Body.* New York, McGraw-Hill, 1975.

BUILDING SKILLS

First aid is the application of principles to situations where people who are ill or injured need immediate help. Knowing the principles of first aid is not sufficient, however. Good emergency caregivers have to be able to think clearly, remember the principles of first aid, and then *do something for the victim.* Being able to do something requires skills. To help insure that the student learns the skills as well as the principles of first aid, specific exercises are included at the end of each chapter in this book. Carefully studying the exercises and carrying out the recommended activities after reading the chapter will help you learn the skills and gain proficiency in first aid.

For each exercise, read over the information given and review the sections of the chapter that apply before carrying out the activities. This practice will help to reinforce the text material while illustrating proper applications of the principles.

I. Emergency care resources in your community

Directions: Catalog the source of emergency care available in your community according to the type of help available. How could you get help from these sources quickly in the event of an emergency?

POLICE/SHERIFF

Official telephone: (day)_____(night)_____(emergency)_____

Services provided: _____

_____

_____

Hours available:_____

Approximate response time to your residence:_____

Cost of services:_____

FIRE DEPARTMENT

Official telephone: (day)_____(night)_____(emergency)_____

Services provided: _____

_____

_____

Hours available:_____

Approximate response time to your residence:_____

Cost of services:_____

AMBULANCE/RESCUE SQUAD

Official telephone: (day)_____(night)_____(emergency)_____

Services provided: _____

_____

_____

Hours available:_____

Approximate response time to your residence:_____

Cost of services:_____

POISON CONTROL CENTER

Official telephone: (day)_____(night)_____(emergency)_____

Services provided: _____

_____

_____

Hours available:_____

Approximate response time to your residence:_____

Cost of services:_____

HOSPITAL(S) WITH EMERGENCY MEDICAL TREATMENT FACILITIES

Hospital and Location:_____

Official telephone: (day)_____(night)_____(emergency)_____

Services provided: _____

_____

_____

Hours available:_____

Approximate response time from your residence:_____

Cost of services:_____

Hospital and Location:_____

Official telephone: (day)_____(night)_____(emergency)_____

Services provided: _____

_____

_____

Hours available:_____

Approximate response time to your residence:_____

Cost of services:_____

OTHER RELATED COMMUNITY SERVICE(S)

Name and Location:_____

Official telephone: (day)_____(night)_____(emergency)_____

Services provided: _____

_____

_____

Hours available:_____

Approximate response time to your residence:_____

Cost of services:_____

II. How the good samaritan law applies to you

Directions: Are your actions as an emergency caregiver controlled by the laws of the state or local government where you live? Find out now.

Briefly outline the major points regarding the laws governing first aid in your community.

a.   Laws governing rendering of first aid

b.   Automobile driver responsibilities

c.   Liabilities for injuries on private property

d.   Definition of negligence

e.   Preferences of local police/sheriff regarding behavior of emergency caregivers at crime scenes

First Steps in Giving Emergency Care: Conducting a Thorough Survey

Assessment of injuries and illnesses is the most important part of first aid. Without accurate assessment, any actions you take in trying to help the victim are likely to be in vain.

The goals of assessment are simple and clear: first, to determine whether the life of the victim is in immediate jeopardy and, second, to investigate injuries and illnesses. Note that diagnosis is not included as a goal. Physicians are responsible for arriving at diagnoses, not emergency caregivers.

In this chapter two types of assessments are discussed: ABC assessment (also called the primary survival scan) and head-to-toe assessment, also known as the secondary survey.

POINTS TO REMEMBER

The **first step** in beginning an assessment is to *try to establish personal contact with the victim* in a way that informs the person of your intentions. If the victim is conscious, introduce yourself and identify yourself as a person with first aid training. These actions will often help to calm the victim and establish your role as rescuer. This communication with the victim will also be helpful to you in beginning your assessment.

Second, always *arrange for additional help* — ambulance, police, fire, etc.—if there is any possibility it will be needed.

Third, always *have a reason for taking action* to help the injured person. If no clear course of action can be justified, then nothing more should be done except to insure that no further injuries occur while more help is en route.

Fourth, *never move a victim without sufficient manpower*, unless it is necessary to protect the person from further injury.

Finally, a quick survey of the circumstances of the victim (see Figure 2-2) will provide clues about how the accident occurred. Do not place complete trust in what you conclude from a quick look, however, because a careful assessment of the victim will provide more evidence that might contradict your original conclusion.

The assessment of an injured or sick individual should be carried out systematically and with great care. The procedures to be used in this process are summarized in Figure 2-1. (This chapter will follow the steps outlined in this figure.)

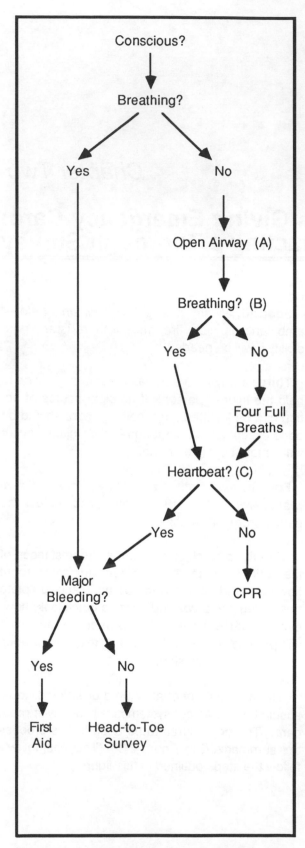

Figure 2-1. *Procedures for Assessment*

Consciousness

The first step in the ABC survey is determining basic consciousness. Basic consciousness is whether the person can respond to sound and gentle touch. To discover consciousness ask in a loud voice "Are you OK?" As you speak, touch the victim on the shoulder and squeeze gently. The combination of these two actions will arouse conscious victims and elicit some form of response. It is important to be gentle in assisting consciousness and avoid rough handling to prevent aggravating undiscovered injuries (such as neck injuries). If the victim speaks, moans, coughs, moves, or gives any visible or audible response, then the ABC survey will be much easier because it is already clear that the victim is breathing and has a heartbeat. If the victim does not respond, the emergency caregiver must proceed quickly and carefully and complete the airway, breathing and circulation steps.

Airway and Breathing

For the unconscious victim in whom breathing and heartbeat are not established, first priority is to determine whether the victim is breathing—if not, then you must begin immediately to correct this problem.

When breathing stops, immediate action is needed (rescue breathing). When heartbeat stops, immediate action is needed (CPR). See chapter 3 for details.

Once breathing stops, it only takes about four minutes for tissue to begin to die. This process is especially rapid in the brain and after four minutes there is a *geometric decrease* in survival rate for each additional minute the brain remains *deoxygenated*. This is due to the fact that the brain cannot store oxygen nor incur *oxygen debt*. A helpful reminder is that if the victim is talking or crying out in pain, then the victim is obviously breathing.

It is essential to remember that further efforts to aid the victim must wait until the airway is opened and the victim is breathing.

20

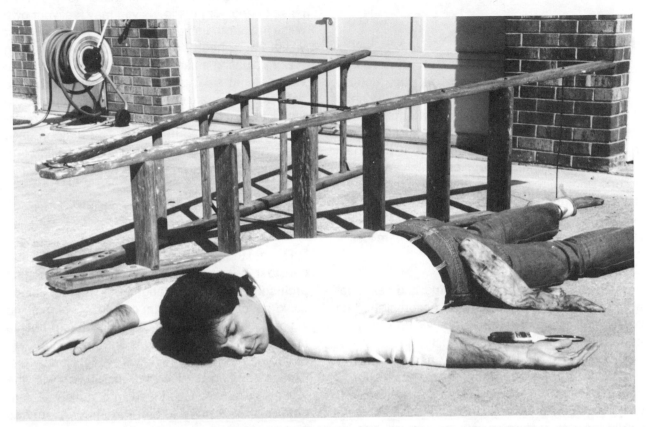

Figure 2-2. *The position of the victim, the victim's clothing, and the surroundings, all provide important clues about how injuries may have occurred.*

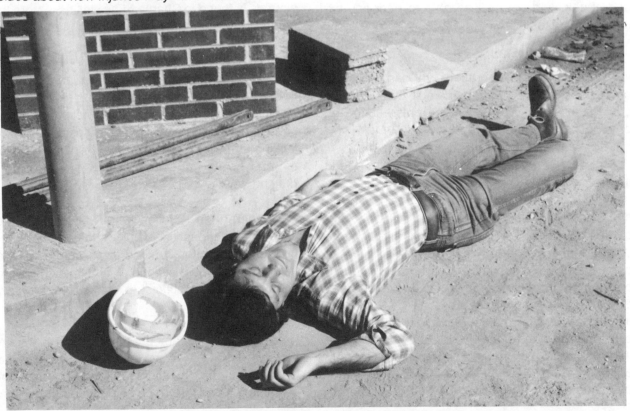

Heartbeat

Once you have checked on the victim's breathing, you should next determine if the heart is beating. It may be found that the victim's breathing has stopped but the heart is still beating. In some cases, both respiration and heartbeat cease. When the heart stops or beats very weakly, organs and systems are no longer receiving oxygen and nutrients. The same critical situation exists concerning lack of oxygen to tissues, whether respiratory or cardiac function (or both) are lost or diminished.

It is best to check both breathing and heartbeat at the same time. This may be accomplished by positioning yourself beside your victim with your knees on either side of the victim's shoulders. Turn your head and put your ear near the victim's mouth as if you were listening for the victim to whisper something to you. From this position, you will be able to see any chest movement which would indicate respiratory effort. You will also be able to feel any exchange of air against your ear and cheek, and you will be able to hear any exchange of gases (See Figure 2-3).

At the same time you are kneeling beside your victim to check for respiration, you can check the pulse as an indicator of cardiac activity. The most convenient place to feel for the pulse during an emergency is at the *carotid artery.*

The carotid pulse may be found by placing the index and middle fingers lightly on the side of the neck. The carotid artery runs just beside the trachea on either side. By gently moving the fingertips downward until a notch is felt, you will be able to feel or *palpate* the pulse located over the carotid artery. When the carotid notch is found, press gently downward until you feel the pulse. You must be careful not to press inward toward the trachea as you may make breathing more difficult or stimulate the *gag reflex.* Depth of compression is important also. If you do not compress deeply enough, a faint pulse may not be felt; if you compress too deeply, the pulse may be closed off.

You should never use your thumb to check the pulse of another person, as you may feel your own pulse in your thumb and wrongly assume that your victim has a heart beat. One additional warning about palpating a carotid pulse—if you are on your victim's right side, take the victim's pulse on the right side; if you are on the left, take the pulse from the victim's left side. If you reach across the victim's trachea to find the pulse, you may produce the same problems as those discussed with compressing the carotid artery inward.

Hemorrhage

The next step in the primary survival scan is to consider hemorrhage. If the victim is bleeding profusely, there is a danger that enough blood could be lost that the victim could die if something is not done to control the bleeding. It is probable that heavy bleeding, which is life threatening, will be arterial. Arterial bleeding is recognized by distinctive spurting of blood that correlates with the victim's pulse. Venous bleeding can also be dangerous if extensive. Life-threatening venous bleeding is associated with other major trauma. A more complete discussion of hemorrhaging wounds is found in Chapter 4 as well as a more indepth discussion of how to determine and control the severity of bleeding.

If the victim is breathing and his heart is beating but he is bleeding heavily, you must stop the flow of blood before you continue. The presence of profuse hemorrhaging will be easily ascertained by looking for pools of blood around or near your victim and noting the characteristics of the hemorrhaging wound.

A general rule to follow when determining the extent and seriousness of blood loss is that anything over one liter of blood in an adult and one half liter in a child is serious. Many times the sight of blood makes it difficult to estimate objectively the quantities lost.

Estimation of the amount of blood lost is important but difficult to do accurately for people who work in emergency settings. One quick means of estimating blood loss is by comparison of pulses.

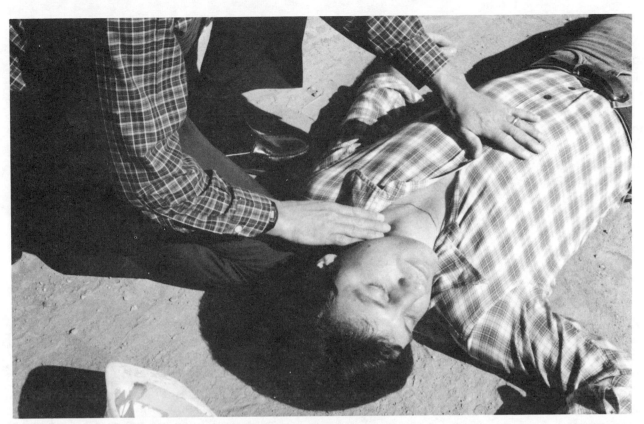

Figure 2-3. *To check breathing and heartbeat, place one hand on the victim's chest and the fingers of the other hand on the carotid artery. Bend down over the victim's mouth and look at the chest so you can hear breathing and watch the chest rise and fall.*

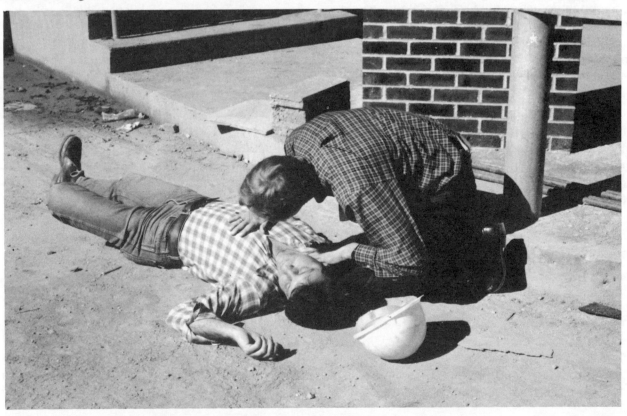

This is an especially good means of estimating internal blood loss where you are unable to see the actual blood. If you are able to feel a carotid pulse, then you know the victim has a systolic blood pressure of > 60 mm/hg. If you have a palpable radial pulse (this pulse is on the wrist on the same side as the thumb), you know the victim's blood pressure is > 80 mm/hg. Then if you find a carotid pulse and no radial pulse, you may assume the loss of 1-2 liters of blood which has caused the drop in blood pressure.

SUMMARY

Now you have completed the ABC survey to identify the three immediate life-threatening emergencies: airway obstruction, cardio-pulmonary arrest and severe hemorrhage. Other conditions may exist which could eventually become life-threatening emergencies. The following section describes a comprehensive head-to-toe search for such injuries.

Before proceeding to the head-to-toe survey, it is important to understand a concept that must remain foremost in dealing with emergency situations. The idea every rescuer must keep in mind is that *proactive* measures reduce the need for "reactive" measures which are more dangerous and less effective. In other words, if you can keep something from happening you are a more efficient and effective rescuer. Proactive refers to monitoring vital signs and symptoms of the victim and doing something about them before they develop into a major problem. Reactive efforts are aimed at doing something about a problem that has already developed. An adequate rescuer is a capable reactive technician while the truly effective rescuer is proactive.

THE HEAD-TO-TOE SURVEY

General Rules

1. Once you have completed the check for responsiveness and have done a primary survival scan, you must make a more detailed examination of the victim. In this phase of emergency care you will attempt to discover any additional injuries needing treatment.

2. If the victim is conscious, you should introduce yourself and explain what you would like to do in order to accomplish this task. With a conscious victim it is critical that you be in command and maintain the confidence of your victim. Confidence is best communicated by knowing what you are doing and explaining everything you do beforehand. If you are clear in explaining your actions, you will promote the cooperation of the victim and others.

3. Know your limits. Perhaps one of the most crucial skills to master in the survey is to realize when the situation at hand calls for competencies you do not possess. The ability to recognize situations beyond your control and scope of training may prove vital to the survival of the victim. To that end, keep in mind the following: If you do not know what you are doing, do nothing, and if you are not sure of how to do something, stop.

4. Be aware of spine and neck injuries. Any unconscious patient should be treated as if there is a spinal injury until proper measures are taken to indicate no such damage exists.

5. Continually monitor the victim for changes. Once you have taken initial vital signs you must continue to monitor for changes.` At regular intervals you must take repeated measures and compare them to the original ones. Many times the changes which occur over time are more indicative of what is happening than the actual initial measures.

Before beginning a head-to-toe survey, review the data you already have. If, for example, you have a victim who is unconscious, breathing, not severely hemorrhaging and suffering from undetermined injuries, the possibility exists that this person may be suffering from spinal injuries. Until determination of the existence of such injuries can be made, it is of critical importance that all moving and handling of the victim be kept at a minimum.

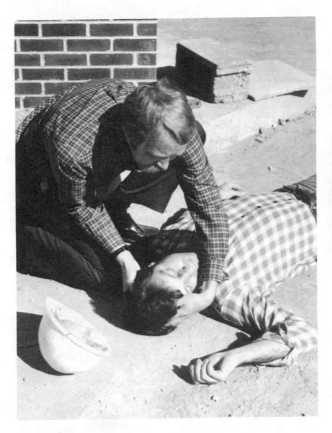
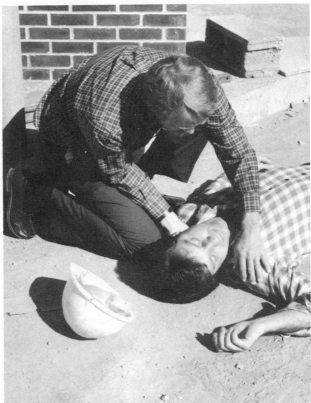

Figure 2-4. *Check the victim's skull and neck* without changing the victim's position. *A good head-to-toe survey is both thorough and systematic.*

Head, Face and Neck

Look for obvious injuries, feel for things which are not as they should be, and finally listen for irregular or unusual sounds. This you will do in a well-defined order, beginning with the head, face and neck.

Very lightly run your fingertips through the victim's hair, covering the entire skull except for that area in contact with the surface on which the victim is lying. Palpate for depressions of the skull, the presence of blood, fresh or clotted masses, or bone fragments. You have not moved the head yet because you do not know if the victim has spinal injuries. Very carefully, without moving the victim's neck, palpate the cervical spine (neck). While palpating the skull and neck, inspect the face for diagnostic signs. First, look for bruises on the face which might indicate blunt trauma. Next, check to see if there are fluids draining from the ear or nose. If there is blood coming from either opening, is it mixed with another clear fluid?

Now observe the pupils of the victim's eyes, looking for several things. First see how the pupils react to light. This person's eyes have been closed and should be *dilated*. When you lift the lids, the pupils should immediately react to the light by *constricting* in an involuntary reaction. If the pupils fail to react, this is an indication that the brain may not be getting enough oxygen for some reason.

Another condition that you may find is that of constricted pupils. Constricted pupils are usually the result of a central nervous system disorder or the abuse of narcotic drugs or stimulants. In either case, something extraordinary has happened to the central nervous system either through illness, trauma or chemicals.

If one pupil reacts to light but the other does not, there are several possible explanations. One explanation would be that the nonresponsive eye is a *prosthesis*. A prosthesis is an artificial replacement for a body part, in this case an artificial eye. Another answer could be that the brain was dam-

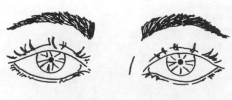

Constricted Pupils

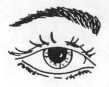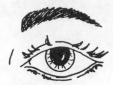

Dilated Pupils

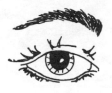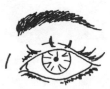

Unequal Pupils

Figure 2-5. *Size of pupils is an important sign of head injury.*

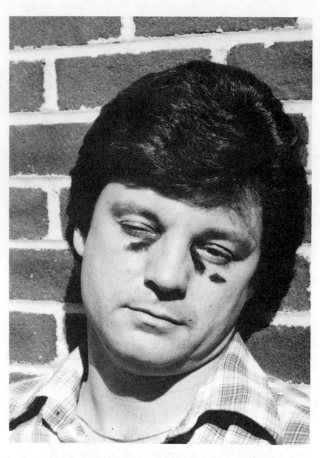

Figure 2-6. *Unusual patterns of bruising are important indicators of injury. Raccoon sign (above), for example, is an indicator of basal skull fracture.*

aged by trauma or *cerebrovascular accident*. Usually one side of the brain is injured and the opposite side of the body is affected. In stroke, this would mean that if a stroke affects the left side of the brain there could be motor problems on the right side of the body. Pupillary reaction in stroke is not necessarily the same. From the eye the optic nerve crosses before it goes to the brain; thus pupil constriction of the left eye could mean injury to the left side of the brain.

It is now time to observe the face for specific signs which will indicate possible head injury. First look for *raccoon sign* (Figure 2-6). Raccoon sign is bruises under both eyes. (The appearance is simi-

lar to the black mask of a raccoon.) The presence of this sign is indicative of a *basal skull fracture*. The basal skull fracture is extremely difficult to diagnose even in the clinical setting with the use of x-ray. Because of the difficulty of diagnosis, anyone with raccoon signs should be treated as if he or she has a skull fracture even in the absence of other symptoms.

Next, look behind and below the ears. The presence of a bruise here is referred to as *Battle's signs* and also indicates skull fracture. Like raccoon signs, Battle's signs should be treated as a definitive diagnosis of skull fracture, even in the absence of other signs and symptoms.

Skin

While observing for the more obvious raccoon and Battle's signs, also observe the general color and texture of the skin. You may notice a bluish tint which marks *cyanosis* of tissue. Cyanosis suggests respiratory distress, lung disease, airway obstruction or impaired cardiac function. This sign normally occurs around the nose, ears, fingernail beds and the lips. The bluish discoloration is indicative of a lack of oxygen getting to the cells of the body. This diagnostic sign indicates a respiratory emergency and demands immediate attention.

A pallor or ashen grey color may point out shock while a flushed skin may be indicative of fever or heat stroke. Notice also if the skin is hot or cool, dry or moist. Skin which is cool and moist is said to be *clammy*.

During the assessment, you may have found an obvious cause for the victim's problem and be able to do something about it right away. On the other hand, you may have discovered the victim's problem and realized that there was really nothing you could do about it. If this is the case, you need to get the victim to medical care.

Central Nervous System

Next, we need to know something about the status of the central nervous system (CNS), especially the spinal cord. In order to make some determination of the CNS system in an unconscious patient we must use pain stimuli. We cannot ask this victim to move arms and legs nor ask questions about numbness. We will be able to make some guesses about CNS involvement as well as the level of consciousness through this technique. If we pinch the soles of the feet or palms of the hands, we will be able to make some determination of the victim's level of consciousness and/or *cerebrospinal* involvement.

If the victim reacts to painful stimuli on one side by withdrawing or making other purposeful movements but does not do so when the other side is stimulated, we may assume that the victim has had a stroke. If the victim moves the arms but not the legs, we should assume some type of spinal cord damage. If the victim moves neither arms nor legs, there may be spinal cord damage or deep coma. It is obvious that if CNS involvement is indicated, all handling of your victim must be minimized in the remainder of your assessment.

If, at this point, you have no reason to suspect neck injuries, you may go back and very carefully move your victim's head to palpate that area in contact with the ground.

Chest: Sternum and Ribs

Assuming the victim has no cerebrospinal injuries, carefully examine the person from the shoulder girdle down.

After completing the assessment of the thorax and shoulder, check the extremities. Check for depressions, protrusions, deformities, tenderness and/or discoloration. Begin by lightly running your fingertips over the clavicle and scapula, humerus, radius and ulna. Look at the wrist, hand and fingers.

When surveying the chest, watch and listen to the breathing process as well as inspect pertinent anatomy. The sternum should be checked for depression and then each rib palpated. While working the thorax, note if the chest is rising equally on both sides. If not, be aware that the victim may soon develop respiratory distress and appropriate action will be needed. If there are respirations but the chest is not rising, the victim is *belly breathing*. While the victim is breathing at the moment, this condition can deteriorate and become life-threatening. As there is inadequate oxygen for normal functioning, over time there may be respiratory failure.

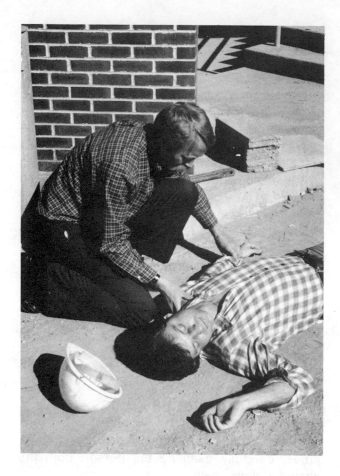
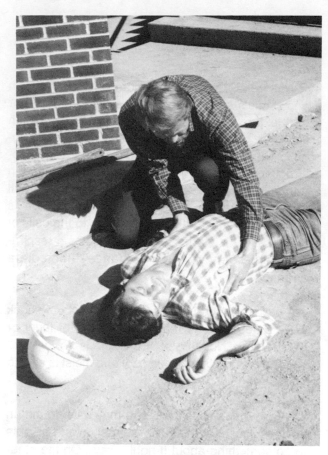

Figure 2-7. *Carefully feel the shoulders, ribs and sternum, checking for deformities and tenderness.*

If on palpation you find that there are depressed areas in the sternum or ribs, be aware of the possibility of breathing complications and be alert for progressively worsening vital signs. An area of ribs where there are three or more ribs fractured in more than one place is referred to as *flail chest*. This is a complicated problem and can be extremely dangerous.

The Abdomen

If there are no respiratory problems, we move on to the abdominal cavity. Palpate each of the four *abdominal quadrants* looking for rigidity, *guarding, tenderness* and/or discoloration. These signs may indicate internal injury or hemorrhage and the presence of any of these signs suggests the need for immediate medical attention. The help needed to correct any inter-abdominal problem is beyond the scope of our training and the victim should be transported to medical care without delay.

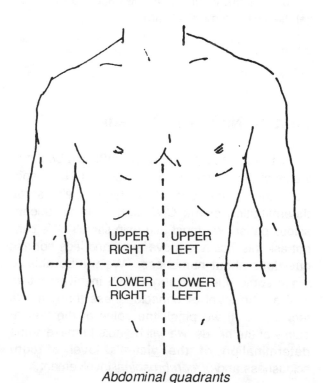

Abdominal quadrants

28

The Pelvis and Hip

If there is nothing to indicate immediate attention in the abdomen, we move on to the pelvis and hip. The next step in the head-to-toe survey is to compress the sides of the pelvis inward. If the victim expresses pain on compression, assume that there is a fractured pelvis. If there are no pelvic problems, move to assess the hip.

To assess the hip for fractures observe the legs. If one leg is turned out, shorter than the other or the muscles are rotated, assume hip fracture in that leg. If the knee on one side is drawn up and the leg is rotated inward, assume dislocation of the hip.

The Lower Extremities

Knee and Kneecap. Palpation of the patella (kneecap) will disclose fractures or dislocations. Fractures are usually the result of blunt trauma. A fractured patella will have a great deal of swelling and discoloration. Pain will be great and the patient will resist attempts to move the leg. In fact, the leg should be treated as it lies and not moved any more than necessary.

Dislocations of the kneecap are easily seen in most cases. The dislocated patella will be displaced to the side of the joint. In the space previously occupied by the patella, there will appear a depression or dip. If there is a dislocated patella, the leg should be immobilized and the joint protected.

Femur. It is often difficult to feel the femur because the quadriceps muscles surrounding this bone are quite large. If the femur is fractured, there will probably be a great deal of swelling which will be easily visible. Also, the fractured femur often results in gross deformity or rotated quadriceps muscles. Finally, the surrounding muscles may be in contraction or the break may be open. In the presence of any of the above signs, determination of the femur fracture is not usually difficult.

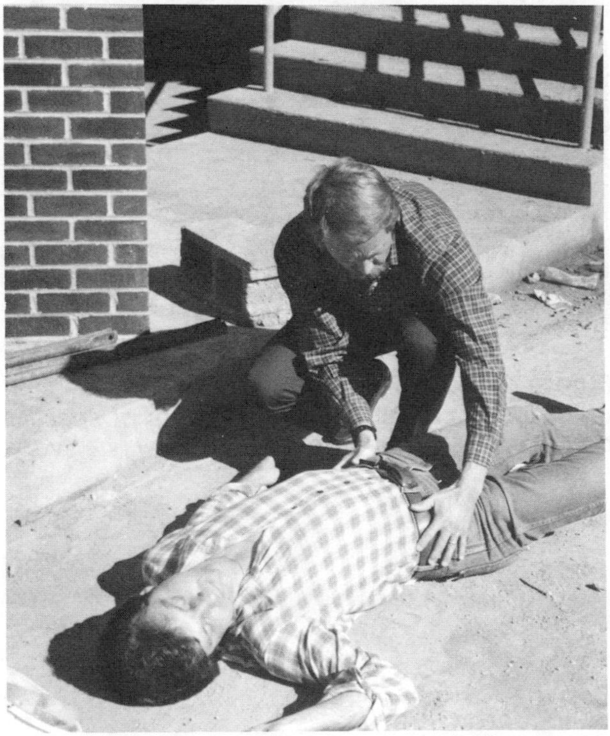

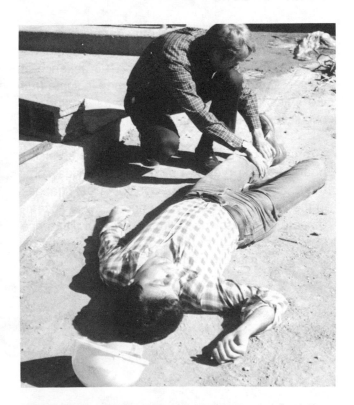

Figure 2-8. *Press the hips together from the sides, using the hands to check for injuries to the pelvic bones.*

Figure 2-9. *Systematically inspect and feel the legs and feet. If in doubt about a deformity, remember that bodies are symmetrical and that left and right should match.*

Tibia/Fibula. In feeling of the lower leg, it is important to remember that many times both the tibia and fibula are broken. Finding one bone broken may not account for all symptoms of a fracture in the lower leg. Be complete in your survey of the lower leg.

Ankle/Foot. It will be difficult to determine the difference between fractures of the foot and sprains and strains of the ankle. The signs and symptoms of both are nearly identical. There will be swelling, discoloration and pain in the affected area. Many times the definitive diagnosis for fracture versus sprain in the foot can be made only by x-ray. Given this difficulty in determination, fractures and sprains should be treated in the same manner. Dislocations of the ankle will be obvious as there will be gross deformity, swelling and pain. In many cases, the outline of the bone ends may be seen in this dislocation.

Final Checks

Once we have completed our search we need to go back and make some more discrete judgments by checking peripheral pulses. The absence of pulses at wrist or foot locations may indicate that we missed a fracture which was cutting off circulation, or that cardiac function is diminishing.

In cases of conscious victims, a comprehensive head-to-toe survey is not so important as communication with the victim. Consider what changes in the head-to-toe survey are necessary to accommodate the conscious victim. The major difference in an assessment for the conscious versus unconscious victim is to whom you speak.

Physically, you will handle the victim the same way and do the same things to find injuries or illness. In the case of an unconscious victim, you ask questions of other people at the scene as to what happened. With a conscious victim, you ask the patient what happened. They will be able to tell you what they saw, heard or felt. You will need to ask them what their chief complaint is or what hurts or bothers them most. It will be important to find out the victim's medical history as it may have an impact on what should be done or what caused the problem. In this type of assessment, you will be able to eliminate many things and depending upon the type of accident and the capability of the victim to provide you with accurate and complete information about his condition and what happened, you may reduce the need for a complete head-to-toe survey.

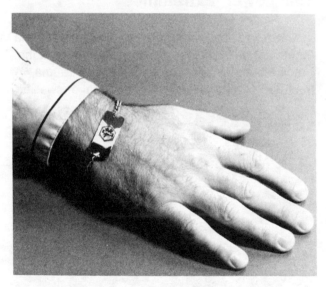

Figure 2-10. *Some victims have necklaces or other identification notifying rescuers of specific conditions. This information may be very important.*

THE HEAD-TO-TOE SURVEY

A. **Begin with the ABCs**

1. Breathing
2. Heart beating
3. Profuse bleeding

B. **Palpate skull and cervical spine without changing victim's position.**

C. **Take note of skin:**
1. Cool, warm or hot
2. Dry, moist or clammy
3. Cyanotic, ashen or cherry red

D. **Check response of pupils:**
1. Fixed
2. Constricted
3. Dilated
4. Uneven

E. **Check nervous system:**
1. Response to deep pain stimuli if appropriate

2. Arms
3. Legs

F. **Go back and finish skull examination.**
1. Dents, bumps, lacerations

G. **Search for fractures of the chest, back, and upper extremities:**
1. Ribs and sternum
2. Chest expansion equal
3. Shoulder girdle
4. Extremities

H. **Palpate abdominal quadrants:**
1. Rigid
2. Guarding
3. Discoloration

I. **Examine pelvis, hip and lower extremities.**

J. **Check peripheral pulses.**

Your ability to make the victim relaxed and confident in you will greatly increase the patient's cooperation. The patient's cooperation in answering questions increases the effectiveness of communication. Communication and cooperation are very important because it is the information gained from the victim that enables you to make a more competent judgment about what is to be done.

SUMMARY

Now you have made a complete head-to-toe survey and noted many signs in the process. Your ability to put all these signs in perspective and make a sound decision will depend partly on how well you master the content in the following chapters. Before moving to specific content, here is an outline of the primary survival scan of the total head-to-toe survey.

BUILDING SKILLS: FIRST STEPS IN GIVING EMERGENCY CARE: CONDUCTING A THOROUGH SURVEY

Assessment skills are basic and essential for the emergency caregiver. However, correct assessment of each body system requires different technical skills, and integrating the information collected is yet another skill. The exercises for this chapter focus on each system individually and culminate in the total survey. Each skill has its own technique, and practice will enable you to carry out the assessment correctly and come to an appropriate conclusion.

Name_____

Directions: Divide into groups of three or more. One student should act as the victim, another student as the emergency caregiver, and the remaining student(s) as observer. Carry out the indicated skill or observation listed for each section (I-VII).

	SKILL OR OBSERVATION	PROFICIENCY	

I. Consciousness

Satisfactory   *Recheck*

a. Correct approach to the victim   _____   _____

b. Attempts to arouse victim without movement   _____   _____

c. "Are you OK?" in a loud voice   _____   _____

d. Sensitivity -—finger/toe touch   _____   _____

e. Other _____   _____   _____

f. Comments on student performance   _____

_____

_____

II. Cardiovascular Assessment

Satisfactory   *Recheck*

a. Check for breathing   _____   _____

b. Open airway if necessary   _____   _____

c. Character of breathing   _____   _____

   rate _____

   depth of respiration _____

   regularity _____

d. Check carotid pulse   _____   _____

e. Character of pulse   _____   _____

   rate/min _____

   regularity _____

SKILL OR OBSERVATION	PROFICIENCY	
	Satisfactory	*Recheck*

Cardiovascular Assessment, *Continued*

f. Peripheral pulses

    radial   _____   _____   _____

    foot   _____

g. Other _____   _____   _____

h. Comments on student performance _____

_____

_____

III. Nervous System Assessment

	Satisfactory	*Recheck*
a. inspect for facial symmetry	_____	_____
b. Sensitivity to touch	_____	_____
c. Grip strength symmetry	_____	_____
d. Symmetry of toe touch against hand	_____	_____
e. Mental status	_____	_____
date and place	_____	_____
birthday	_____	_____
address/telephone	_____	_____
correct recent memory	_____	_____
f. Other _____	_____	_____

    Comments on student performance _____

_____

_____

Name_____

SKILL OR OBSERVATION	PROFICIENCY	
	Satisfactory	*Recheck*

IV. Bones and joints

a. Palpation of limb with joint   _____   _____

b. Systematic examination   _____   _____

c. Check for symmetry of body halves   _____   _____

d. Other deformities surveyed   _____   _____

e. Other _____   _____   _____

f. Comments on student performance _____

_____

_____

V. Skin

                                          Satisfactory   *Recheck*

a. Color   _____   _____

b. texture—wet/dry   _____   _____

c. temperature   _____   _____

d. Other _____   _____   _____

e. Comments on student performance _____

_____

_____

VI. Eyes

                                          Satisfactory   *Recheck*

a. Pupils

     dilated/constricted   _____   _____

     equality   _____   _____

     reactive to light   _____   _____

b. Vacant/engaged   _____   _____

VII. Putting all the parts together

Directions: Now that you've had a chance to practice all the components of the assessment, you need to put the parts together and carry out an assessment. Following the steps shown below, carry out the assessment and note your findings.

a. ABC survey _____

　　Respiration _____

　　Heartrate _____

　　Bleeding (yes/no) _____

b. Recheck consciousness _____

_____

c. Scalp and head

　　lacerations, dents and bumps _____

_____

　　eyes _____

　　ears and nose _____

d. Neck and cervical spine _____

e. Shoulders, arms and hands _____

_____

f. Chest and sternum _____

g. Abdomen _____

h. Pelvis _____

i. Legs _____

j. Feet _____

k. Other _____

Comments on Student Performance _____

_____

_____

Chapter Three

Insuring Respiration and Heartbeat: Rescue Breathing and CPR

In Chapter 2, the ABC survey was presented as the most basic operation of emergency caregivers. Recall that "A" is for airway, "B" for breathing and "C" for circulation (heartbeat). These three items are the basis for emergency care in this chapter as well. This chapter will build on the ABC survey and present the procedures for dealing with emergencies involving airway, breathing and circulation.

Respiration (breathing) and heartbeat are the two most basic prerequisites for life. Interruption of either will end life promptly. Emergency caregivers, therefore, must have a clear understanding of what can and should be done to preserve and/or restore breathing and heartbeat. Since the procedures for emergency care for breathing and heartbeat are somewhat complex, this chapter is organized around the steps put forth in Figure 3-1. This figure depicts a logical series of steps that are part of the care needed to maintain life. It will be helpful to the reader to periodically refer to the figure to help maintain a sense of the logical progression of procedures presented.

> The best way to become comfortable with artificial respiration and CPR is to complete a formal course in the subject. Check with the American Red Cross or the American Heart Association

RESPIRATION

All processes of the living cell are dependent on an adequate supply of oxygen to carry on normal functioning. Respiration is the process whereby living tissues use oxygen. If enough cells die, the victim dies.

Oxygen enters the blood through the process of breathing. Breathing is controlled by the central nervous system (CNS) and is an unconscious activity. The CNS is triggered to cause breathing when the levels of carbon dioxide in the blood become elevated. The more carbon dioxide present in the blood, the faster one breathes and vice versa. Any injury, illness or drug action which affects the CNS may therefore affect breathing.

The heart, like the brain, is very oxygen-sensitive and needs an adequate blood supply to carry on normal functioning. The heart may cease to function gradually over time or it may stop working suddenly.

Consciousness

As you recall from Chapter 2, consciousness is one of the first things to be established in a victim.

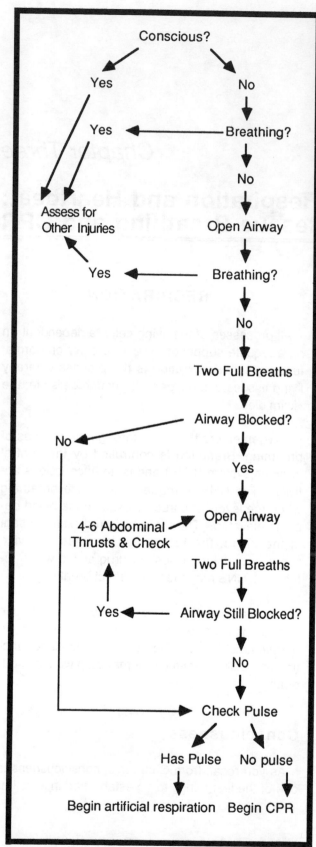

Figure 3-1. *A system for determining consciousness, breathing and heartbeat.*

Gently tap the victim, taking care not to shake the victim and make injuries worse. In a loud voice, ask the victim, "Are you okay?" If the victim is conscious, continue the assessment and determine the nature and extent of the injuries. If there is no response and the victim appears unconscious, the next step is to check for breathing.

Place your face near the victim's mouth and nose, and check for breathing. Place your hand on the victim's chest to check for rising and falling. Listen for the passage of air. Carry out these procedures without moving the victim's head or neck. If the victim is breathing on his own, there is no need to change position. *Remember: always act to prevent injury. An unconscious victim may have a serious neck or spinal injury that may be made worse by improper handling.* If the victim is not breathing, then the next step is to open the airway as soon as possible!

Non-breathing victims may have a closed airway because of their position, or because of a foreign body. Obstruction of the airway due to position is the result of some body part or tissue blocking the airway and is called *anatomical obstruction*. Most commonly, the obstruction is by the tongue or epiglottis.

Opening the Airway

Victims who are unconscious and lying on their backs with no respiration may be suffering from an anatomical obstruction. If the victim's tongue falls back it may block the passage of air into the trachea. Normally the base of the tongue is held in place by the muscles under the tongue. When one is conscious, the muscles of the throat aid in holding the tongue out of the airway. When one loses consciousness, these muscles relax, the *gag reflex* is suppressed, and the tongue may fall backward into the airway.

No matter the age of the victim or the cause of the obstruction, the result is consistent and predictable. If the airway is not opened promptly the victim loses consciousness, the brain loses its

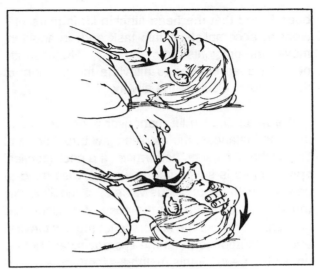

Figure 3-3. *Opening the airway:* ***Top,*** *obstruction of airway is produced by the tongue and epiglottis;* ***Bottom,*** *the obstruction is relieved by head-tilt/chin-lift.*

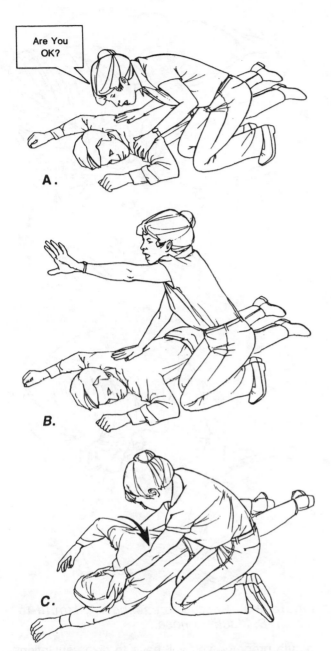

A.

B.

C.

Figure 3-2. *Initial steps of cardiopulmonary resuscitation:* ***A,*** *Determining unresponsiveness;* ***B,*** *Calling for help;* ***C,*** *Positioning the victim.*

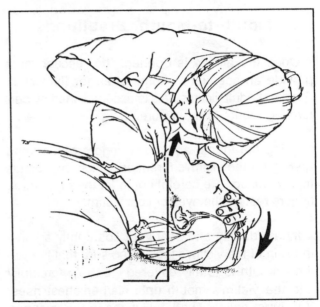

Figure 3-4. *Determining breathlessness.*

supply of oxygenated blood, and automatic impulses to breathe cease. Eventually the heart stops beating and death occurs. Remember that four to six minutes after the victim ceases breathing, brain damage begins. *Biological death* occurs between six and ten minutes after brain tissue is deprived of oxygen.

To open the airway, tilt the victim's head back and lift the chin; this normally moves the tongue and epiglottis out of the airway and alleviates the obstruction. Many people learned cardiopulmonary resuscitation (CPR) a few years ago when the head tilt-neck lift was taught as a means of moving the tongue out of the airway. It has now been found that the head tilt-chin lift is more efficient at accomplishing this task and, in addition, moves the epiglottis out of the way. The head tilt-neck lift does nothing to alleviate the problem of the epiglottis blocking the airway.

The head tilt-chin lift maneuver is preferred but, in some instances, the modified jaw thrust or head tilt-jaw thrust must be performed. If a neck (cervical spine) injury is suspected (always a wise thing to consider with unconscious victims), a modified jaw thrust must be used. In the case of a suspected cervical injury, use the fingers to jut the jaw forward and the thumbs to push the lips downward but do not tilt the head. If this method is ineffective, place the fingers behind the angle of the jaw and push forward. Tilt the head back and push the lower lip downward with your thumbs.

Mouth-to-Mouth Breathing

Once the airway is opened, the rescuer must provide an adequate volume of air for the victim. For most adult victims, this is accomplished by performing mouth-to-mouth breathing.

Using the thumb and index fingers of the hand resting on the victim's forehead, pinch the nostrils tightly closed. Be careful not to let the other three fingers rest on the eyes of your victim.

Inhale deeply and seal your lips tightly against the skin of the victim's face being sure that the victim's mouth is totally covered. Exhale forcefully into the victim's mouth until his/her chest rises. You must deliver two ventilations in this manner, with each ventilation lasting between one to one and one-half seconds. Now, deliver at least one breath every five seconds or twelve per minute until the victim begins to breathe spontaneously.

Mouth-to-Nose

If your victim has loose-fitting dentures, a laceration of the cheek, or some other unusual situation which causes you to not be able to seal the

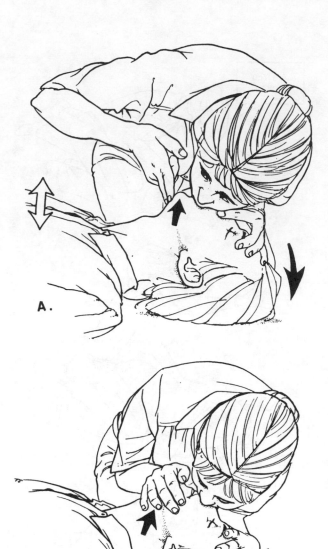

Figure 3-5. *Rescue breathing.* **A,** *Mouth-to-mouth;* **B,** *Mouth-to-nose.*

mouth properly, you will have to give ventilations using the mouth-to-nose technique.

You must maintain the same head tilt that was used in mouth-to-mouth respiration. However, be sure to seal the lips of the victim so that air will not escape. This may be accomplished by using your cheek or the thumb of the hand holding the chin (Fig. 3-5). The mouth is opened wide and sealed completely against the skin of the victim surrounding the nose, and ventilations are given in the same manner as for mouth-to-mouth.

Infants and Children

If the victim is an infant or child, several factors must be taken into consideration for mouth-to-mouth breathing. First is the matter of size. In addition to overall anatomy, the capacity of lungs is less and the air passages are much smaller in infants and children. Second, the anatomy of infants and small children is such that improper technique will actually close off the airway rather than opening it.

In opening the airway of infants, a slight head tilt/chin lift or jaw thrust maneuver will open the airway. Overtilting will close off the airway. In most instances, where foreign body obstruction is not involved, inability to inflate the lungs of infants and small children is due to poor position (Figure 3-6).

For infants, cover the mouth *and* nose with your mouth for mouth-to-mouth breathing. For older children, cover the mouth with your mouth and use your cheek to close off the nose. Procedures for larger children should be the same as for adults.

Adjust the volume of air blown in just so that the chest rises and falls. Take special care to avoid blowing too hard, as serious injury can result.

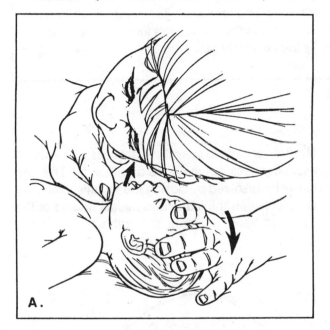

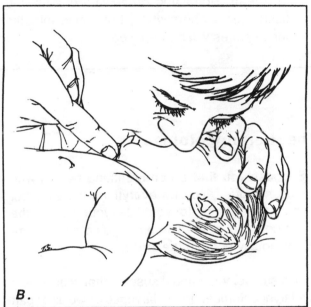

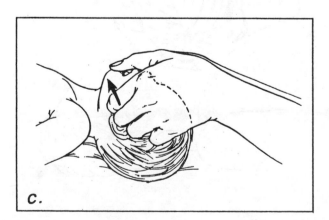

Figure 3-6. *Opening the airway of infants: **A,** Head-tilt/chin-lift; **B,** Jaw-thrust; **C,** Mouth-to-mouth and nose seal.*

Artificial Respiration Works

When spontaneous breathing has stopped, the immediate concern, after opening the airway, is to return an adequate supply of oxygen to the lungs and blood. Once breathing has stopped, the heart can continue beating for several minutes. Existing stores of oxygen will be sufficient to meet the needs of the heart, brain and other vital organs and tissue for a short while, but within minutes these stores will be depleted.

Breathing air inhaled from your lungs into the lungs of another will provide adequate oxygen to maintain life until professional medical care can be obtained. In comparison, the composition of inhaled air — 20% oxygen and 80% nitrogen and exhaled air — 16% oxygen, 34% carbon dioxide and 80% nitrogen—we find roughly three times more oxygen exhaled than used by the body. Thus there is three times more oxygen in exhaled air than the amount needed to support life. It is apparent that the problem in artificial respiration is not the air entering the victim's lungs so much as it is the *volume* of air.

The Laryngectomee

Suppose you find a non-breathing person who is unconscious. You do everything correctly but when you attempt to ventilate your victim, the chest does not rise. The air is going somewhere but obviously not into the lungs.

In this case, you should suspect that your patient is a laryngectomee. In the laryngectomee all or part of the larynx has been removed and there is a *stoma* in the trachea. The laryngectomee breathes partially through the mouth and nose but mostly through the stoma. If you attempt to ventilate a victim with this condition through mouth-to-mouth ventilation, the air passes out of the trachea through the stoma before it gets to the lungs. For the laryngectomee, you need only remove debris from the stoma and seal the mouth tightly over the opening. Head tilt/chin lift is not necessary because the airway opening is below any anatomical obstructions (see Figure 3-7).

When you attempt to ventilate the stoma of a laryngectomee, it is possible that your ventilations will not be resisted and yet the lungs will not rise. In this instance, you might suspect that there is a tube from the stoma to the base of the tongue to

allow for enhanced speech. In this case, air may be escaping back out the nose and mouth. This can easily be resolved by closing the nostrils; pinch the nose between the index and middle fingers of the superior hand and use the palm to cover the mouth.

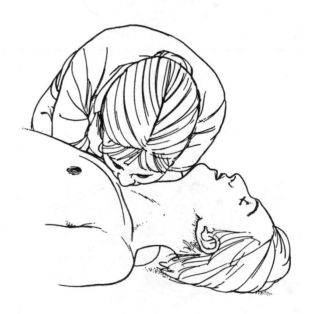

Figure 3-7. *Mouth-to stoma ventilation.*

42

OBSTRUCTION FROM A FOREIGN BODY

A recent report from the American Red Cross indicates that around 3,000 people a year die as a result of airway obstruction. This ranks as the sixth leading cause of accidental death in the United States. Death from choking, otherwise known as "cafe coronary," a significant problem in all age groups, can be treated if recognized early and if effective measures are used to treat the condition.

It seems odd that someone could choke to death in a restaurant and others assume he or she has had a heart attack. Let us examine what happens by considering the hypothetical case history of a person with a "cafe coronary."

An individual is enjoying a meal and has had a few drinks before or with dinner. He ingests a particularly large piece of food which becomes lodged in back of the throat blocking the airway. The person stops eating and talking because no air is moving in or out, and often the victim cannot cough. Soon the individual collapses and may suffer a cardiac arrest from the airway obstruction.

Although many things may play a part in this obstructed airway, the two most frequently recurring factors are alcohol and a large piece of food. Other factors which may contribute to the problem are loose-fitting or missing dentures, missing teeth, or anything which may make effective chewing difficult. Running, exercising, or talking while eating may also be reasons for airway obstruction.

Conscious Victims

A victim who is conscious of airway obstruction will make the problem known. Typically, the person reacts by grasping the throat or pointing to the mouth to alert the rescuer to the problem. If the victim cannot speak or cough, or if there is a high-pitched shrill whistling sound on attempted inspiration, the obstruction is complete.

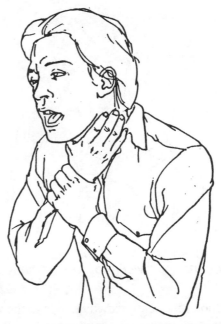

Figure 3-8. *The universal distress signal for foreign body obstruction of the airway.*

Ask the victim, "Are you choking?" If the victim can speak, cough or exhibits signs of exchanging air effectively, the obstruction is incomplete. In the case of an incomplete obstruction, monitor the victim closely but do nothing to the victim.

The involuntary act of coughing will be more effective at relieving the obstruction than anything you can do. In fact, you may make the situation worse by trying to remove the object. Once the victim is no longer able to cough or speak, however, the obstruction is complete and immediate first aid is needed.

First Aid

It is possible that the act of coughing may not relieve the obstructed airway. It is also possible that the victim will eventually cease effective ventilatory efforts. If this is the case, the rescuer must do something to control the situation.

When it is clear that the victim's own efforts are not working, attempt to dislodge the obstruction using abdominal thrusts. With your chest against your victim's back, put your arms under the victim's

43

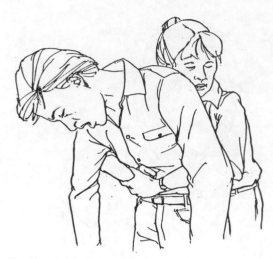

Figure 3-9. *Administering the Heimlich maneuver to a conscious victim of foreign body airway obstruction.*

arms. Choose a point midway between the xiphoid and umbilicus, make a fist, and place it on this midpoint. Grasp the fist with your knuckles pointing up and drive it in and up in a rocking motion. Deliver six to ten quick forceful thrusts. Each thrust should be forceful enough to dislodge the object and should each be distinct from the preceding attempt. If unsuccessful, abdominal thrusts should be repeated until successful or until the victim becomes unconscious. If the victim loses consciousness, the sequence for unconscious victims should begin and continue until successful.

When abdominal thrusts are used to remove airway obstruction, there is a good chance that vomiting will follow. The rescuer then must remain alert to the danger of aspiration of vomitus (inhaling vomitus into the lungs) and take appropriate measures to guard against this happening. Roll the unconscious victim onto his/her side and place in the coma position. If the victim vomits, be sure the face points to the side or downward. After vomiting has stopped, be certain that the airway is clear.

> **Heimlich Maneuver.** The Heimlich Maneuver, popularized by Dr. Henry Heimlich, is a means of dislodging objects that are stuck in the windpipe. By exerting a sudden force on the abdomen, air pressure builds quickly within the respiratory system. This pressure is often sufficient to move the object and allow the victim to breathe.

The victim of an airway obstruction who is alone may self-administer abdominal thrusts. The victim may use his/her own fist to deliver thrusts in the same place as described earlier for conscious victims. The victim may also bend over a chair or other stable object and provide inward and upward pressure against the diaphragm. Pointed or sharp objects should not be used, and positioning of the thrusts must be correct.

First Aid for Unconscious Victims

The first step in providing first aid for airway obstruction is detecting the problem. Once the problem is identified as an airway obstruction caused by a foreign body, the following steps should be taken.

1. Open the airway and try to give breaths.

2. If resistance is felt (no air will go in), go through the "opening-the-airway" steps and try the breaths again. The attempts at breathing should take between one to one and one-half seconds for each breath. Each breath should be sufficient to make the chest rise. If the airway is still blocked, proceed to Step 3.

3. Perform six to ten abdominal thrusts. These thrusts may be delivered from a position beside the victim's hip or straddling the victim. It might be easier to keep your line of compression straight if you straddle the victim. The straddle is the recommended position for rescuers who are physically small or for anyone dealing with a very large victim.

In performing the abdominal thrusts, choose a spot midway between the *xiphoid process* and the *umbilicus* and place the heel of one hand here. The other hand is placed on top and the fingers locked. Now quickly and forcefully deliver four thrusts inward, toward the spine, and upward toward the diaphragm. This will put pressure against the diaphragm which will push against the lungs and force air trapped in the lungs against the obstruction. If this pressure is sufficient, the obstruction will be blown into the upper pharnyx where it can be reached with the fingers.

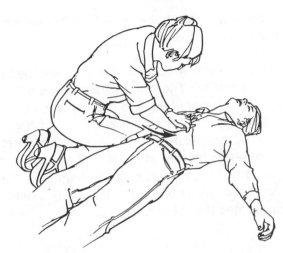

Figure 3-10. *Administering the Heimlich maneuver to an unconscious victim of foreign body airway obstruction.*

4. After the abdominal thrusts, it is possible that the foreign body lodged in the airway may now be accessible. You should therefore begin finger sweeps of the airway. Open the victim's mouth and move the index finger along the inside of the victim's cheek to the back of the airway, feeling for foreign bodies. Care must be taken not to push the foreign object back into the airway during finger sweeps.

If the object cannot be removed, continue the series of opening the airway, ventilation, abdominal thrusts and finger sweeps until you are successful, until more competent help arrives, or the person is declared dead by a physician.

SPECIAL CONSIDERATIONS

Obese and Pregnant Victims. Abdominal thrusts may not be successful in the case of the obese victim, as it would be too difficult to put sufficient pressure against the diaphragm. In the case of pregnant victims, it is dangerous as well as ineffective to use the Heimlich maneuver.

In these instances, the chest thrust is substituted for the abdominal thrust. The chest thrust is carried out by wrapping the arms around the individual, making a fist (as for the abdominal thrust) and applying sharp pressure to the mid sternum (breast bone).

Infants and Children. Children account for approximately one-fourth of deaths from airway obstruction each year. Most of these obstructions are from objects the child places in the mouth, such as parts of toys, bottle caps, burst balloons or anything of interest on the floor.

Check for responsiveness by tapping the shoulder gently, or with infants, flip the sole of the foot. If the child is unconscious, open the airway and attempt to give breaths. If efforts are resisted, reposition and try again. If unsuccessful, give four chest thrusts. *(Do not use abdominal thrusts on children.)* Attempt to see the foreign body by using the tongue lift-jaw lift maneuver. If the object cannot be seen, attempt to give breaths again. Repeat this sequence until successful.

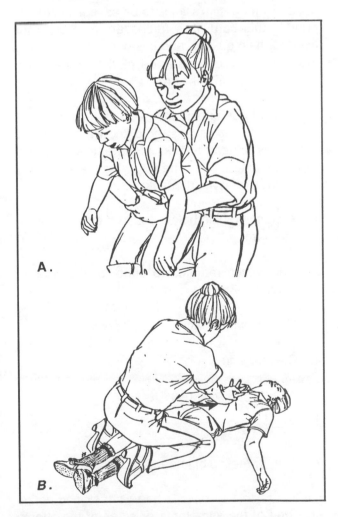

Figure 3-11. *Administering the Heimlich maneuver to a child:* **A,** *with child standing;* **B,** *with child lying.*

CARDIOPULMONARY CIRCULATION

Heart Attack/Sudden Death

The functioning of the heart is controlled in large part by the brain. If the brain ceases to function, the heart will stop. If the heart gradually weakens it is generally the result of chronic disease. If the heart stops suddenly it is often because the blood supply has been interrupted to part of the heart. Sudden cessation of heart beat is usually referred to as cardiac arrest. Cardiac arrest which results in death before help can arrive is referred to as sudden death.

When the heart stops beating, immediate care is needed if the victim's life is to be saved. In order to provide this care, it is necessary to assess the need for help quickly, and it is of equal importance that the rescuer be trained in the proper techniques to provide this care.

In order to determine the need for intervention in heart attack, it is necessary to know the signs and symptoms of heart attack. Heart attack often precedes cardiac arrest. The following are symptoms of an impending heart attack:

1. A crushing pain below and in the middle of the sternum.

2. Pain which radiates to either of the arms or jaws.

3. Nausea with or without vomiting

4. Clammy skin

5. A feeling of weakness

6. Cyanosis

7. Fear or feeling of impending doom

It is possible to have a heart attack and notice only one of the symptoms or signs of the attack. The more signs and symptoms present and the stronger the symptoms, the more likely it is the victim is having a heart attack.

Many times the symptoms of *angina* and heart attack are similar. The major differences are that angina pain is over in three to five minutes and is generally related to physical exertion or emotional stress. The pain related to heart attack is constant and is generally unrelieved by rest. After the onset of symptoms of heart attack, the average delay in seeking treatment is one to two hours. This delay is many times the sole cause of death from heart attack.

If the victim is suffering from an angina attack, the person should be moved to a resting position. If the victim has medication it should be delivered as prescribed.

If you suspect a heart attack, follow these steps:

1. Under no circumstances should the patient be allowed to assist you in moving.

2. Place the victim in a semi-reclining position.

3. Loosen restrictive clothing.

4. Try to create an atmosphere of calm relaxation as much as possible.

5. Activate the EMS system.

6. Constantly monitor vital signs.

The Unconscious Victim of Cardiac Arrest

The need for cardiopulmonary resuscitation (CPR) is discovered once you have begun to administer artificial respiration. You discover your victim does not have a carotid pulse. This you determine as part of the ABC survey . (A full discussion of the patient survey is found in Chapter 2.) When you have checked the carotid pulse for a full five to ten seconds and find no signs of a heartbeat, you must begin CPR.

CPR is a lifesaving technique which artificially moves blood to the the vital organs (brain, heart, and lungs) by externally compressing the chest. If the chest were open, we could hold the heart in our hands and squeeze, sending blood out of the *ventricles*, or pumping chambers. Of course, this is not generally possible, but the same compression of the heart can be accomplished in a different way.

If the chest can be compressed correctly, blood will be forced out of the ventricles and into the vessels supplying the heart, lungs and brain. Research has shown that when the chest is compressed during CPR, all valves in the heart remain open. It is as a result of this finding that the compression phase of CPR has been changed from 60 to 80 compressions per minute. This is discussed in detail later in this section.

As blood is forced out of the heart into a closed and filled system, then blood will be forced back into the heart. Adequately ventilating the victim while artificially moving the blood is the process of cardiopulmonary resuscitation (CPR).

First Aid

In considering CPR, most people think of the physical skills necessary to oxygenate and move the blood. In fact, these skills are only the second most important predictor of survival in cardiac arrest. The most critical factor seems to be how soon advanced help is available to the victim. This fact illustrates the importance of getting professional help for heart attack victims.

The second critical factor in survival is the time delay between the attack and the beginning of CPR. The longer the time between the attack and institution of life support measures, the less the chance of survival of the victim. While advanced help is critical, basic skills may keep the victim alive until advanced life support help arrives.

After you have activated the EMS system, the victim must be placed on a firm surface. If the sur-

face below the victim is soft, then the force of cardiac compressions will be absorbed without compressing the thoracic cavity. Placing the victim on the floor is a perfectly acceptable placement for the administration of CPR.

The rescuer's position in relation to the victim is the same as that for artificial resuscitation. The rescuer should kneel beside the victim with knees on either side of the victim's shoulders. From this position the rescuer should be able to move rapidly from chest compressions to ventilations and back again with a minimum of time loss and movement.

Correctly position the hands on the victim's chest. This is done by finding the xiphoid process, a cartilage protrusion at the end of the sternum. A depression at the distal end of the sternum marks the location of the xiphoid. Place the index and middle finger of the hand closest to the feet of the victim, on the xiphoid. With the hand closest to the victim's head, place the heel of the hand on the sternum while touching the fingers covering the xiphoid. Now place the inferior hand on top of the hand on the sternum. Lock the fingers so that only the heel of the superior hand is in contact with the skin (Figure 3-12).

Compression of the sternum is accomplished by leaning directly over the victim with locked elbows transferring weight to the hands. When the sternum is compressed, the shoulders of the rescuer should be directly over the hands and the elbows should be locked. Compress the sternum vertically one and one-half to two inches for an adult victim. During the relaxation phase of the compression/relaxation cycle, the hands should not lose contact with the skin of the chest. This will insure that the hands remain in the correct position for compressions. The skin-to-skin contact with the chest must be maintained and, at the same time, all pressure must be released so that the heart will be allowed to refill completely. The rescuer should deliver between 60 to 80 compressions per minute. However, it is essential that the rescuer not be so concerned with the rate that the quality of compressions is overlooked.

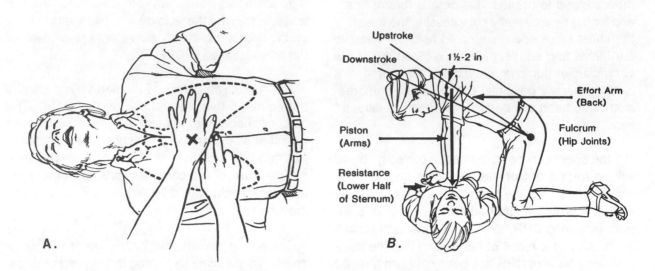

Figure 3-12. *External chest compression: **A,** locating the correct hand position; **B,** proper position of the rescuer, with shoulders directly over the victim's sternum and the elbows locked.*

Traditionally, a rate of 60 compressions per minute has been recommended for one-rescuer CPR with each compression lasting for 50% of the compression/relaxation cycle. In practice, more attention seems to be directed to complying with the rate criteria. Rescuers may meticulously count off one per second cardiac compressions, often without concentrating on whether they maintain each compression for the required amount of time. In fact, duration of compression is a more important variable to control than is the number of compressions performed per minute.

By increasing the compression rate to 80 per minute, the total time of compressions is reduced, thus making it easier to achieve the 50% compression/relaxation cycle.

Once CPR has been started, it should not be interrupted for more than five seconds to check for return of pulse and reaction of pupils to light. CPR may be interrupted for 15-30 seconds in order to move the victim when transportation becomes a necessity. Any unnecessary interruption of CPR results in the heart, lungs, and brain doing without oxygen. Survival is at this point critical.

Summary: One Rescuer CPR

The following is an outline of the steps used in administration of CPR:

1. Establish lack of responsiveness and open the airway.
2. Give the victim two breaths.
3. Check for the carotid pulse.
4. If there is no pulse, activate the emergency system.
5. Compress the chest 15 times. (These compressions should be slightly faster than one per second or 60-80 per minute.)
6. Ventilate the victim twice. (Ventilations should be between .8 and 2.0 liters of air each.)
7. Continue to alternate 15 compressions and 2 ventilations until you are successful or until more qualified help arrives to replace you.
8. Re-check for the return of carotid pulse after four cycles of fifteen compressions or approximately one minute. Continue the cycle and re-check every eight to ten cycles or two minutes after.

The training of basic rescuers in two-person CPR has been deleted. Procedures for switching between compressions and ventilations were too cumbersome and difficult to master. In addition, the physical skills necessary for successful two-rescuer resuscitation deteriorate very rapidly if not practiced regularly. Few non-professionals have the time or access to equipment to maintain physical skills; therefore a month after initial training they would be ineffective at two rescuer resuscitation. The American Heart Association now reserves this type of training for qualified emergency and medical personnel only.

For rescuers at the basic level of training the following is the recommended procedure for treatment of cardiac arrest with two rescuers.

Cardiopulmonary Resuscitation with Two Rescuers

1. One rescuer is performing CPR alone.
2. A second rescuer arrives, assumes a position at the head of the victim, and identifies him/herself as trained in CPR and willing to assist.
3. The second rescuer finds a carotid pulse which is generated from cardiac compression and looks for the chest to rise in order to assess the effectiveness of CPR.
4. When help is requested by the first rescuer, two ventilations are given and CPR terminated.
5. Now the second rescuer checks for a carotid pulse for five seconds.
6. If there is no pulse, the second rescuer gives two ventilations.
7. The second rescuer continues CPR at the normal rate and ratio.
8. The first rescuer continually assesses the adequacy of the second rescuer's ventilations and compressions.
9. This is continued until successful or until better trained help becomes available.

Gastric Distention

All rescuers must be aware that no matter how conscientious the rescuer is in performance of CPR, there may be a bypass of air which is forced into the stomach instead of the lungs. This was especially true under the old "four quick breaths" guidelines. The longer CPR is performed, the greater the chance this will occur. When air is forced into the trachea through artificial respiration, some of it will be forced into the esophagus and eventually the stomach. When this bypass occurs, there will be a noticeable increase in the size of the stomach. This is referred to as *gastric distention*.

Gastric distention means the stomach is filling with air. This is important for two reasons. First, if the stomach swells enough it may pressure the diaphragm and thus compromise the ability to ventilate the victim. Secondly, gastric distention will usually terminate with the victim *vomiting*. A victim on his back who vomits may *aspirate* the contents of the stomach. Aspiration is inhaling fluids or vomit into the lungs. Aspiration of stomach contents often results in a form of chemical pneumonia which is extremely difficult to treat and is often fatal.

Do not treat gastric distention unless it interferes with your ability to ventilate the victim. Treatment for gastric distention is as follows:

1. First roll the victim on his/her side.
2. Press firmly in the middle of the abdomen.
3. Be prepared to clean the victim's airway, as relieving gastric distention usually results in vomiting.
4. After the airway has been cleared, roll the victim over on the back and resume CPR.

Figure 3-13. *Treating gastric distention:* **A,** *reposition the airway;* **B,** *exert moderate pressure on the abdomen.*

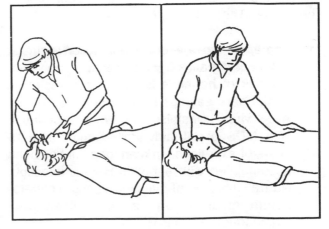

Infants and Children

Infants vary slightly in the requirements for CPR. First the proper place to check for a pulse in an infant is the brachial artery. The carotid may be difficult to find and the area over the heart may indicate pre-cardiac (impulse) activity and not true (pulse-blood flow) heartbeats. Secondly, an infant is compressed near mid-sternum between 1/2 to 1 inches, using the index and middle fingers of one hand. In order to find the correct compression point for an infant, draw a line across the nipples and down the sternum. The point of compression is one finger's width below the intersection of this imaginary line.

Finally, the infant is compressed at a rate between 90-100 times per minute. A special warning for doing CPR on a flat surface with infants: when an infant's head is hyperextended, the infant's shoulders will rise off of the surface. Thus, compressions may do damage. In this case, you should pad the space between the shoulders of the infant so placed.

Children require less depth of compression to provide adequate artificial circulation. In fact, excessive compression depth may be harmful to children, doing damage to underlying structures and organs. The sternum of a child should be compressed only one to one-half inches. The compression rate is slightly faster for children than for adults. The compression rate for children is 80-90 per minute.

Treatment Procedure

1. Check for responsiveness.
2. Open airway and check for breath.
3. If no breathing give two ventilations lasting one to one and one half seconds each.
4. Check brachial pulse.
5. Activate the emergency system.
6. Give chest compressions one finger width below a line drawn across the nipples and down the sternum.
7. Compress the sternum 1/2 to 1 inches at a rate of 90 to 100 per minute.
8. Give one ventilation after each five compressions.

> **Take a CPR course. The local office of the American Red Cross or American Heart Association can help you.**

Mouth-to-Mouth and Acquired Immunodeficiency Syndrome (AIDS)

You should understand the AIDS virus and its transmission before making a decision about performing or withholding mouth-to-mouth rescue breathing. These are the facts:

1. The *epidemiology* of AIDS infection is similar to that of hepatitis B virus infection. However, the risk of hepatitis B virus transmission in health care settings far exceeds that for the AIDS virus transmission. While experience with AIDS is still fairly limited, more than 15 years of experience in management has been accumulated with hepatitis B virus infection. No transmission of infection during mouth-to-mouth resuscitation has ever been documented for hepatitis B.

2. Though final answers are not in, the potential risk of transmission of AIDS by mouth-to-mouth resuscitation appears to be extremely small.

The final point to consider in this question is this: If you do not perform rescue breathing for a victim who needs it, the victim will die of hypoxia whether or not he or she has AIDS.

The authors wish to give special thanks to Dr. Ken Grauer and Dr. Larry Kravitz of the University of Florida Medical College for their permission to use the information related to AIDS. These data are a partial result of their extensive work in cardiac management.

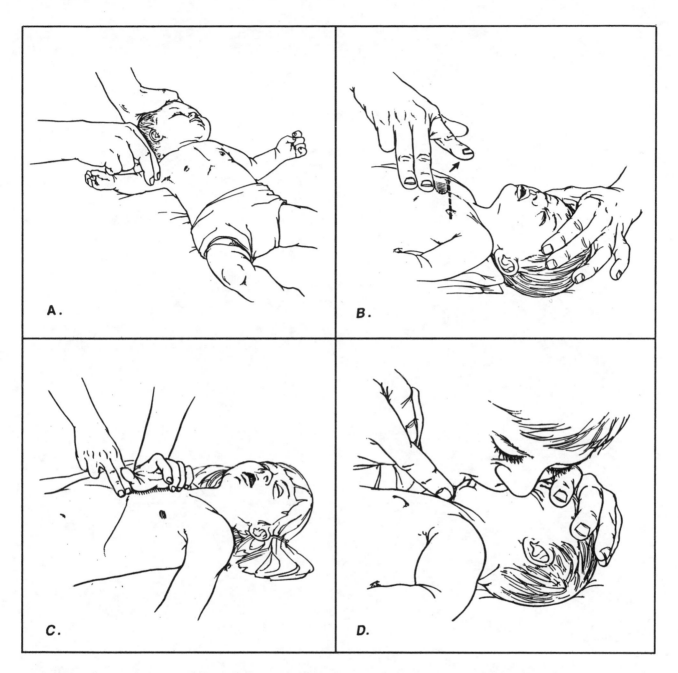

Figure 3-14. *Performing CPR with children and infants: **A,** locating and palpating the brachial pulse; **B,** locating hand position for chest compressions in children; **C,** locating the finger position for chest compressions in infants; **D,** Mouth-to-mouth and nose seal.*

Further Readings

M. Levy, M. Dignan, J. Sherreffs: *Life and Health,* 5th Edition, New York, Random House, 1987. Chapter 14, "Cardiovascular Health and Disease."

USDHSS, PHS, CDC: Recommendations for Prevention of HIV Transmission in Health-Care Settings. *Morbidity and Mortality Weekly Report* (Supplement), Vol. 36, No. 2S, August 21, 1987.

BUILDING SKILLS: CHAPTER THREE

Skills for restoring breathing and heartbeat are taught as a unit in CPR (Cardio-Pulmonary Respiration) and BLS (Basic Life Support) courses. To avoid confusion, skill sheets recommended by the American Heart Association are included here to guide you in gaining proficiency in resuscitation procedures.

Obstructed Airway: Conscious Adult

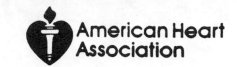

American Heart Association

Name _____ Date _____

Step	Activity	Critical Performance	S	U
1. Assessment	Determine airway obstruction.	Ask "Are you choking?"		
		Determine if victim can cough or speak.		
2. Heimlich Maneuver	Perform abdominal thrusts.	Stand behind the victim.		
		Wrap arms around victim's waist.		
		Make a fist with one hand and place the thumb side against victim's abdomen in the midline slightly above the navel and well below the tip of the xiphoid.		
		Grasp fist with the other hand.		
		Press into the victim's abdomen with quick upward thrusts.		
		Each thrust should be distinct and delivered with the intent of relieving the airway obstruction.		
		Repeat thrusts until either the foreign body is expelled or the victim becomes unconsious (see below).		

Victim with Obstructed Airway Becomes Unconscious (Optional Testing Sequence)

Step	Activity	Critical Performance	S	U
3. Additional Assessment	Position the victim.	Turn on back as unit.		
		Place face up, arms by side.		
	Call for help.	Call out "Help!" or, if others respond, activate EMS system.		
4. Foreign Body Check	Perform finger sweep.*	Keep victim's face up.		
		Use tongue-jaw lift to open mouth.		
		Sweep deeply into mouth to remove foreign body.		
5. Breathing Attempt	Attempt ventilation (airway is obstructed).	Open airway with head-tilt/chin-lift.		
		Seal mouth and nose properly.		
		Attempt to ventilate.		
6. Heimlich Maneuver	Perform abdominal thrusts.	Straddle victim's thighs.		
		Place heel of one hand against victim's abdomen, in the midline slightly above the navel and well below the tip of the xiphoid.		
		Place second hand directly on top of first hand.		
		Press into the abdomen with quick upward thrusts.		
		Perform 6–10 abdominal thrusts.		
7. Foreign Body Check	Perform finger sweep.*	Keep victim's face up.		
		Use tongue-jaw lift to open mouth.		
		Sweep deeply into mouth to remove foreign body.		
8. Breathing Attempt	Attempt ventilation.	Open airway with head-tilt/chin-lift.		
		Seal mouth and nose properly.		
		Attempt to ventilate.		
9. Sequencing	Repeat sequence.	Repeat Steps 6–8 until successful.†		

* During practice and testing, simulate finger sweeps.

† After airway obstruction is removed, check for pulse and breathing. (a) If pulse is absent, ventilate a second time and start cycles of compressions and ventilations. (b) If pulse is present, open airway and check for spontaneous breathing. (c) If breathing is present, monitor breathing and pulse closely, maintain open airway. (d) If breathing is absent, perform rescue breathing at 12 times/min and monitor pulse.

Instructor _____ Check: Satisfactory _____ Unsatisfactory _____

4/86

55

Obstructed Airway: Conscious Child*

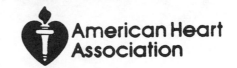
American Heart Association

Name _____ Date _____

Step	Activity	Critical Performance	S	U
1. Assessment	Determine airway obstruction.*	Ask "Are you choking?"		
		Determine if victim can cough or speak.		
2. Heimlich Maneuver	Perform abdominal thrusts (only if victim's cough is ineffective and there is increasing respiratory difficulty).	Stand behind the victim.		
		Wrap arms around victim's waist.		
		Make a fist with one hand and place the thumb side against victim's abdomen, in the midline slightly above the navel and well below the tip of the xiphoid.		
		Grasp fist with the other hand.		
		Press into the victim's abdomen with quick upward thrusts.		
		Each thrust should be distinct and delivered with the intent of relieving the airway obstruction.		
		Repeat thrusts until either the foreign body is expelled or the victim becomes unconsious (see below).		

Victim with Obstructed Airway Becomes Unconscious (Optional Testing Sequence)

Step	Activity	Critical Performance	S	U
3. Additional Assessment	Position the victim.	Turn on back as unit.		
		Place face up, arms by side.		
	Call for help.	Call out "Help!" or if others respond, activate EMS system.		
4. Foreign Body Check	Perform tongue-jaw lift. Do not perform blind finger sweep; remove foreign body only IF VISUALIZED.	Keep victim's face up.		
		Use tongue-jaw lift to open mouth.		
		Look into mouth and remove foreign body IF VISUALIZED.		
5. Breathing Attempt	Attempt ventilation (airway is obstructed).	Open airway with head-tilt/chin-lift.		
		Seal mouth and nose properly.		
		Attempt to ventilate.		
6. Heimlich Maneuver	Perform abdominal thrusts.	Kneel at victim's feet if on the floor, or stand at victim's feet if on a table.		
		Place heel of one hand against victim's abdomen, in the midline slightly above navel and well below tip of xiphoid.		
		Place second hand directly on top of first hand.		
		Press into the abdomen with quick upward thrusts.		
		Perform 6–10 abdominal thrusts.		
7. Foreign Body Check	Perform tongue-jaw lift: Do not perform blind finger sweep; remove foreign body only IF VISUALIZED.	Keep victim's face up.		
		Use tongue-jaw lift to open mouth.		
		Look into mouth and remove foreign body IF VISUALIZED.		
8. Breathing Attempt	Attempt ventilation.	Open airway with head-tilt/chin-lift.		
		Seal mouth and nose properly.		
		Attempt to ventilate.		
9. Sequencing	Repeat sequence.	Repeat Steps 6–8 until successful.†		

* This procedure should be initiated in a conscious child only if the airway obstruction is due to a witnessed or strongly suspected aspiration and if respiratory difficulty is increasing and the cough is ineffective. If obstruction is caused by airway swelling due to infection such as epiglottitis or croup, these procedures may be harmful; the child should be rushed to the nearest ALS facility, allowing the child to maintain the position of maximum comfort.

† After airway obstruction is removed, check for pulse and breathing. (a) If pulse is absent, ventilate a second time and start cycles of compressions and ventilations. (b) If pulse is present, open airway and check for spontaneous breathing. (c) If breathing is present, monitor breathing and pulse closely and maintain an open airway. (d) If breathing is absent, perform rescue breathing at 15 times/min and monitor pulse.

Instructor _____ Check: Satisfactory _____ Unsatisfactory _____

4/86

Obstructed Airway: Conscious Infant*

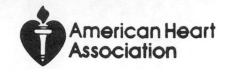
American Heart Association

Name _____ Date _____

Step	Activity	Critical Performance	S	U
1. Assessment	Determine airway obstruction.*	Observe breathing difficulties.*		
2. Back Blows	Deliver 4 back blows.	Supporting head and neck with one hand, straddle infant face down, head lower than trunk, over your forearm supported on your thigh.		
		Deliver 4 back blows, forcefully, between the shoulder blades with the heel of the hand (3–5 sec).		
3. Chest Thrusts	Deliver 4 chest thrusts.	While supporting the head, sandwich infant between your hands and turn on back, with head lower than trunk.		
		Deliver 4 thrusts in the midsternal region in the same manner as external chest compressions, but at a slower rate (3–5 sec).		
4. Sequencing	Repeat sequence.	Repeat Steps 2 and 3 until either the foreign body is expelled or the infant becomes unconscious (see below).		

Infant with Obstructed Airway Becomes Unconscious (Optional Testing Sequence)

Step	Activity	Critical Performance	S	U
5. Call for Help.	Call for help.	Call out "Help!" or, if others respond, activate EMS system.		
6. Foreign Body Check	Perform tongue-jaw lift. Do not perform blind finger sweep; remove foreign body only IF VISUALIZED.	Do tongue-jaw lift by placing thumb in infant's mouth over tongue. Lift tongue and jaw forward with fingers wrapped around lower jaw.		
		Remove foreign body IF VISUALIZED.		
7. Breathing Attempt	Attempt ventilation (airway is obstructed).	Open airway with head-tilt/chin-lift.		
		Seal mouth and nose properly.		
		Attempt to ventilate.		
8. Back Blows	Deliver 4 back blows.	Supporting head and neck with one hand, straddle infant face down, head lower than trunk, over your forearm supported on your thigh.		
		Deliver 4 back blows, forcefully, between the shoulder blades with the heel of the hand (3–5 sec).		
9. Chest Thrusts	Deliver 4 chest thrusts.	While supporting the head and neck, sandwich infant between your hands and turn on back, with head lower than trunk.		
		Deliver 4 thrusts in the midsternal region in the same manner as external chest compressions, but at a slower rate (3–5 sec).		
10. Foreign Body Check	Perform tongue-jaw lift, not blind finger sweep.	Do tongue-jaw lift.		
		Remove foreign body IF VISUALIZED.		
11. Breathing Attempt	Reattempt ventilation.	Open airway with head-tilt/chin-lift.		
		Seal mouth and nose properly.		
		Attempt to ventilate.		
12. Sequencing	Repeat sequence.	Repeat Steps 8–11 until successful.†		

* This procedure should be initiated in a conscious infant only if the airway obstruction is due to a witnessed or strongly suspected aspiration and if respiratory difficulty is increasing and the cough is ineffective. If the obstruction is caused by airway swelling due to infections, such as epiglottitis or croup, these procedures may be harmful; the infant should be rushed to the nearest ALS facility, allowing the infant to maintain the position of maximum comfort.

† After airway obstruction is removed, check for breathing and pulse. (a) If pulse is absent, ventilate a second time and start cycles of compressions and ventilations. (b) If pulse is present, open airway and check for spontaneous breathing. (c) If breathing is present, monitor breathing and pulse closely and maintain an open airway. (d) If breathing is absent, perform rescue breathing at 20 times/min and monitor pulse.

Instructor _____ Check: Satisfactory _____ Unsatisfactory _____

Obstructed Airway: Unconscious Adult

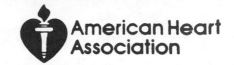

American Heart Association

Name _____ Date _____

Step	Activity	Critical Performance	S	U
1. Assessment/Airway	Determine unresponsiveness.	Tap or gently shake shoulder. Shout "Are you OK?"		
	Call for help.	Call out "Help!"		
	Position the victim.	Turn on back as unit, if necessary, supporting head and neck (4–10 sec).		
	Open the airway.	Use head-tilt/chin-lift maneuver.		
	Determine breathlessness.	Maintain open airway.		
		Ear over mouth, observe chest: look, listen, feel for breathing (3–5 sec).		
2. Breathing Attempt	Attempt ventilation (airway is obstructed).	Maintain open airway.		
		Seal mouth and nose properly.		
		Attempt to ventilate.		
	Reattempt ventilation (airway remains blocked).	Reposition victim's head.		
		Seal mouth and nose properly.		
		Reattempt to ventilate.		
	Activate EMS system.	If someone responded to call for help, send him/her to activate EMS system.		
		Total time, Steps 1 and 2: 15–35 sec.		
3. Heimlich Maneuver	Perform abdominal thrusts.	Straddle victim's thighs.		
		Place heel of one hand against victim's abdomen in the midline slightly above the navel and well below the tip of the xiphoid.		
		Place second hand directly on top of first hand.		
		Press into the abdomen with quick upward thrusts.		
		Each thrust should be distinct and delivered with the intent of relieving the airway obstruction.		
		Perform 6–10 abdominal thrusts.		
4. Foreign Body Check	Perform finger sweep.*	Keep victim's face up.		
		Use tongue-jaw lift to open mouth.		
		Sweep deeply into mouth to remove foreign body.		
5. Breathing Attempt	Attempt ventilation.	Open airway with head-tilt/chin-lift maneuver.		
		Seal mouth and nose properly.		
		Attempt to ventilate.		
6. Sequencing	Repeat sequence.	Repeat Steps 3–5 until successful.†		

* During practice and testing simulate finger sweeps.

† After airway obstruction is removed, check again for pulse and breathing. (a) If pulse is absent, ventilate a second time and start cycles of compressions and ventilations. (b) If pulse is present, open airway and check for spontaneous breathing. (c) If breathing is present, monitor breathing and pulse closely, maintain open airway. (d) If breathing is absent, perform rescue breathing at 12 times/min and monitor pulse.

Instructor _____ Check: Satisfactory _____ Unsatisfactory _____

4/86

Obstructed Airway: Unconscious Child

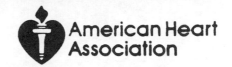
American Heart Association

Name _____ Date _____

Step	Activity	Critical Performance	S	U
1. Assessment/Airway	Determine unresponsiveness.	Tap or gently shake shoulder.		
		Shout "Are you OK?"		
	Call for help.	Call out "Help!"		
	Position the victim.	Turn on back as unit, if necessary, supporting head and neck (4–10 sec).		
	Open the airway.	Use head-tilt/chin-lift maneuver.		
	Determine breathlessness.	Maintain open airway.		
		Ear over mouth, observe chest: look, listen, feel for breathing (3–5 sec).		
2. Breathing Attempt	Attempt ventilation (airway is obstructed).	Maintain open airway.		
		Seal mouth and nose properly.		
		Attempt to ventilate.		
	Reattempt ventilation (airway remains blocked).	Reposition victim's head.		
		Seal mouth and nose properly.		
		Reattempt to ventilate.		
	Activate EMS system.	If someone responded to call for help, send him/her to activate EMS system.		
		Total time, Steps 1 and 2: 15–35 sec.		
3. Heimlich Maneuver	Perform abdominal thrusts.	Kneel at victim's feet if on the floor, or stand at victim's feet if on a table.		
		Place heel of one hand against victim's abdomen in the midline slightly above navel and well below tip of xiphoid.		
		Place second hand directly on top of first hand.		
		Press into the abdomen with quick upward thrusts.		
		Each thrust should be distinct and delivered with the intent of relieving the airway.		
		Perform 6–10 abdominal thrusts.		
4. Foreign Body Check	Perform tongue-jaw lift. Do not perform blind finger sweep; remove foreign body only IF VISUALIZED.	Keep victim's face up.		
		Use tongue-jaw lift to open mouth.		
		Look into mouth and remove foreign body IF VISUALIZED.		
5. Breathing Attempt	Reattempt ventilation.	Open airway with head-tilt/chin-lift maneuver.		
		Seal mouth and nose properly.		
		Attempt to ventilate.		
6. Sequencing	Repeat sequence.	Repeat Steps 3–5 until successful.*		

* After airway obstruction is removed, check for pulse and breathing. (a) If pulse is absent, ventilate a second time and start cycles of compressions and ventilations. (b) If pulse is present, open airway and check for spontaneous breathing. (c) If breathing is present, monitor breathing and pulse closely and maintain an open airway. (d) If breathing is absent, perform rescue breathing at 15 times/min and monitor pulse.

Instructor _____ Check: Satisfactory _____ Unsatisfactory _____

4/86

Obstructed Airway: Unconscious Infant

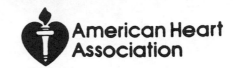
American Heart
Association

Name _____ Date _____

Step	Activity	Critical Performance	S	U
1. Assessment/Airway	Determine unresponsiveness.	Tap or gently shake shoulder.		
	Call for help.	Call out "Help!"		
	Position the infant.	Turn on back as unit, if necessary, supporting head and neck.		
		Place on firm, hard surface.		
	Open the airway.	Use head-tilt/chin-lift maneuver to sniffing or neutral position.		
		Do not overextend the head.		
	Determine breathlessness.	Maintain open airway.		
		Ear over mouth, observe chest: look, listen, feel for breathing (3–5 sec).		
2. Breathing Attempt	Attempt ventilation (airway is obstructed).	Maintain open airway.		
		Make tight seal on mouth and nose of infant with rescuer's mouth.		
		Attempt to ventilate.		
	Reattempt ventilation (airway remains blocked).	Reposition infant's head.		
		Seal mouth and nose properly.		
		Reattempt to ventilate.		
	Activate EMS system	If someone responded to call for help, send him/her to activate EMS system.		
		Total time, Steps 1 and 2: 10–25 sec.		
3. Back Blows	Deliver 4 back blows.	Supporting head and neck with one hand, straddle infant face down, head lower than trunk, over your forearm supported on your thigh.		
		Deliver 4 back blows, forecefully, between the shoulder blades with the heel of the hand (3–5 sec).		
4. Chest Thrusts	Deliver 4 chest thrusts.	While supporting the head and neck, sandwich infant between your hands and turn on back, with head lower than trunk.		
		Deliver 4 thrusts in the midsternal region in the same manner as external chest compressions, but at a slower rate (3–5 sec).		
5. Foreign Body Check	Perform tongue-jaw lift. Do not perform blind finger sweep; remove foreign body only IF VISUALIZED.	Do tongue-jaw lift by placing thumb in infant's mouth over tongue. Lift tongue and jaw forward with fingers wrapped around lower jaw.		
		Remove foreign body IF VISUALIZED.		
6. Breathing Attempt	Reattempt ventilation.	Open airway with head-tilt/chin-lift.		
		Seal mouth and nose properly.		
		Attempt to ventilate.		
7. Sequencing	Repeat sequence.	Repeat Steps 3–6 until successful.*		

*After airway obstruction is removed, check for breathing and pulse. (a) If pulse is absent, ventilate a second time and start cycles of compressions and ventilations. (b) If pulse is present, open airway and check for spontaneous breathing. (c) If breathing is present, monitor breathing and pulse closely and maintain an open airway. (d) If breathing is absent, perform rescue breathing at 20 times/min and monitor pulse.

Instructor _____ Check: Satisfactory _____ Unsatisfactory _____

4/86

CPR and ECC Performance Sheet
One-Rescuer CPR: Adult

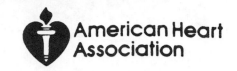

Name _____ Date _____

Step	Activity	Critical Performance	S	U
1. Airway	Assessment: Determine unresponsiveness.	Tap or gently shake shoulder.		
		Shout "Are you OK?"		
	Call for help.	Call out "Help!"		
	Position the victim.	Turn on back as unit, if necessary, supporting head and neck (4–10 sec).		
	Open the airway.	Use head-tilt/chin-lift maneuver.		
2. Breathing	Assessment: Determine breathlessness.	Maintain open airway.		
		Ear over mouth, observe chest: look, listen, feel for breathing (3–5 sec).		
	Ventilate twice.	Maintain open airway.		
		Seal mouth and nose properly.		
		Ventilate 2 times at 1–1.5 sec/inspiration.		
		Observe chest rise (adequate ventilation volume.)		
		Allow deflation between breaths.		
3. Circulation	Assessment: Determine pulselessness.	Feel for carotid pulse on near side of victim (5–10 sec).		
		Maintain head-tilt with other hand.		
	Activate EMS system.	If someone responded to call for help, send him/her to activate EMS system.		
		Total time, Step 1—Activate EMS system: 15–35 sec.		
	Begin chest compressions.	Rescuer kneels by victim's shoulders.		
		Landmark check prior to hand placement.		
		Proper hand position throughout.		
		Rescuer's shoulders over victim's sternum.		
		Equal compression–relaxation.		
		Compress 1 1/2 to 2 inches.		
		Keep hands on sternum during upstroke.		
		Complete chest relaxation on upstroke.		
		Say any helpful mnemonic.		
		Compression rate: 80–100/min (15 per 9–11 sec).		
4. Compression/Ventilation Cycles	Do 4 cycles of 15 compressions and 2 ventilations.	Proper compression/ventilation ratio: 15 compressions to 2 ventilations per cycle.		
		Observe chest rise: 1–1.5 sec/inspiration; 4 cycles/52–73 sec.		
5. Reassessment*	Determine pulselessness. (If no pulse: Step 6.)†	Feel for carotid pulse (5 sec).		
6. Continue CPR	Ventilate twice.	Ventilate 2 times.		
		Observe chest rise; 1–1.5 sec/inspiration.		
	Resume compression/ventilation cycles.	Feel for carotid pulse every few minutes.		

* 2nd rescuer arrives to replace 1st rescuer: (a) 2nd rescuer identifies self by saying "I know CPR. Can I help?" (b) 2nd rescuer then does pulse check in Step 5 and continues with Step 6. (During practice and testing only one rescuer actually ventilates the manikin. The 2nd rescuer simulates ventilation.) (c) 1st rescuer assesses the adequacy of 2nd rescuer's CPR by observing chest rise during ventilations and by checking the pulse during chest compressions.

† If pulse is present, open airway and check for spontaneous breathing: (a) If breathing is present, maintain open airway and monitor pulse and breathing. (b) If breathing is absent, perform rescue breathing at 12 times/min and monitor pulse.

Instructor _____ Check: Satisfactory _____ Unsatisfactory _____

4/86

67

One-Rescuer CPR: Child*

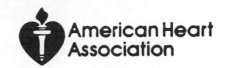
American Heart
Association

Name _____ Date _____

Step	Activity	Critical Performance	S	U
1. Airway	Assessment: Determine unresponsiveness.	Tap or gently shake shoulder.		
		Shout "Are you OK?"		
	Call for help.	Call out "Help!"		
	Position the victim.	Turn on back as unit, if necessary, supporting head and neck (4–10 sec).		
	Open the airway.	Use head-tilt/chin-lift maneuver.		
2. Breathing	Assessment: Determine breathlessness.	Maintain open airway.		
		Ear over mouth, observe chest: look, listen, feel for breathing (3–5 sec).		
	Ventilate twice.	Maintain open airway.		
		Seal mouth and nose properly.		
		Ventilate 2 times at 1–1.5 sec/inspiration.		
		Observe chest rise.		
		Allow deflation between breaths.		
3. Circulation	Assessment: Determine pulselessness.	Feel for carotid pulse on near side of victim (5–10 sec).		
		Maintain head-tilt with other hand.		
	Activate EMS system.	If someone responded to call for help, send him/her to activate EMS system.		
		Total time, Step 1—Activate EMS system:15–35 sec.		
	Begin chest compressions.	Rescuer kneels by victim's shoulders.		
		Landmark check prior to initial hand placement.		
		Proper hand position throughout.		
		Rescuer's shoulders over victim's sternum.		
		Equal compression–relaxation.		
		Compress 1 to 1 1/2 inches.		
		Keep hands on sternum during upstroke.		
		Complete chest relaxation on upstroke.		
		Say any helpful mnemonic.		
		Compression rate: 80–100/min (5 per 3–4 sec).		
4. Compression/Ventilation Cycles	Do 10 cycles of 5 compressions and 1 ventilation.	Proper compression/ventilation ratio: 5 compressions to 1 slow ventilation per cycle.		
		Observe chest rise, 1–1.5 sec/inspiration (10 cycles/60–87 sec).		
5. Reassessment†	Determine pulselessness. (If no pulse: Step 6.)‡	Feel for carotid pulse (5 sec).		
6. Continue CPR	Ventilate once.	Ventilate one time.		
		Observe chest rise; 1–1.5 sec/inspiration.		
	Resume compression/ventilation cycles	Palpate carotid pulse every few minutes.		

* If child is above age of approximately 8 years, the method for adults should be used.

† 2nd rescuer arrives to replace 1st rescuer: (a) 2nd rescuer identifies self by saying "I know CPR. Can I help?" (b) 2nd rescuer then does pulse check in Step 5 and continues with Step 6. (During practice and testing only one rescuer actually ventilates the manikin. The 2nd rescuer simulates ventilation.) (c) 1st rescuer assesses the adequacy of

2nd rescuer's CPR by observing chest rise during ventilations and by checking the pulse during chest compressions.

‡ If pulse is present, open airway and check for spontaneous breathing. (a) If breathing is present, maintain open airway and monitor breathing and pulse. (b) If breathing is absent, perform rescue breathing at 15 times/min and monitor pulse.

Instructor _____ Check: Satisfactory _____ Unsatisfactory _____

4/86

One Rescuer CPR: Infant

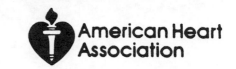

American Heart
Association

Name _____ Date _____

Step	Activity	Critical Performance	S	U
1. Airway	Assessment: Determine unresponsiveness.	Tap or gently shake shoulder.		
	Call for help.	Call out "Help!"		
	Position the infant.	Turn on back as unit, supporting head and neck.		
		Place on firm, hard surface.		
	Open the airway.	Use head-tilt/chin-lift maneuver to sniffing or neutral position.		
		Do not overextend the head.		
2. Breathing	Assessment: Determine breathlessness.	Maintain open airway.		
		Ear over mouth, observe chest: look, listen, feel for breathing (3–5 sec).		
	Ventilate twice.	Maintain open airway.		
		Make tight seal on infant's mouth and nose with rescuer's mouth.		
		Ventilate 2 times, 1–1.5 sec/inspiration.		
		Observe chest rise.		
		Allow deflation between breaths.		
3. Circulation	Assessment: Determine pulse-lessness.	Feel for brachial pulse (5–10 sec).		
		Maintain head-tilt with other hand.		
	Activate EMS system.	If someone responded to call for help, send him/her to activate EMS system.		
		Total time, Step 1–Activate EMS system: 15–35 sec.		
	Begin chest compressions.	Draw imaginary line between nipples.		
		Place 2–3 fingers on sternum, 1 finger's width below imaginary line.		
		Equal compression-relaxation.		
		Compress vertically, 1/2 to 1 inches.		
		Keep fingers on sternum during upstroke.		
		Complete chest relaxation on upstroke.		
		Say any helpful mnemonic.		
		Compression rate: at least 100/min (5 in 3 sec or less).		
4. Compression/Ventilation Cycles	Do 10 cycles of 5 compressions and 1 ventilation.	Proper compression/ventilation ratio: 5 compressions to 1 slow ventilation per cycle.		
		Pause for ventilation.		
		Observe chest rise: 1–1.5 sec/inspiration; 10 cycles/45 sec or less.		
5. Reassessment	Determine pulselessness. (If no pulse: Step 6.)*	Feel for brachial pulse (5 sec).		
6. Continue CPR	Ventilate once.	Ventilate 1 time.		
		Observe chest rise; 1–1.5 sec/inspiration.		
	Resume compression/ventilation cycles.	Feel for brachial pulse every few minutes.		

* If pulse is present, open airway and check for spontaneous breathing.
  (a) If breathing is present, maintain open airway and monitor breathing
and pulse. (b) If breathing is absent, perform rescue breathing at 20 times/min and monitor pulse.

Instructor _____ Check: Satisfactory _____ Unsatisfactory _____

CPR and ECC Performance Sheet
Two-Rescuer CPR: Adult*

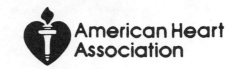

American Heart Association

Name _____ Date _____

Step	Activity	Critical Performance	S	U
1. Airway	One rescuer (ventilator): Assessment: Determines unresponsiveness.	Tap or gently shake shoulder.		
		Shout "Are you OK?"		
	Positions the victim.	Turn on back if necessary (4–10 sec).		
	Opens the airway.	Use a proper technique to open airway.		
2. Breathing	Assessment: Determines breathlessness.	Look, listen and feel (3–5 sec).		
	Ventilator ventilates twice.	Observe chest rise: 1–1.5 sec/inspiration.		
3. Circulation	Assessment: Determines pulselessness.	Palpate carotid pulse (5–10 sec).		
	States assessment results.	Say "No pulse."		
	Other rescuer (compressor): Gets into position for compressions.	Hands, shoulders in correct position.		
	Locates landmark notch.	Landmark check.		
4. Compression/Ventilation Cycles	Compressor begins chest compressions.	Correct ratio compressions/ventilations: 5/1.		
		Compression rate: 80–100/min (5 compressions/3–4 sec).		
		Say any helpful mnemonic.		
		Stop compressing for each ventilation.		
	Ventilator ventilates after every 5th compression and checks compression effectiveness.	Ventilate 1 time (1–1.5 sec). Check pulse to assess compressions.		
	(Minimum of 10 cycles.)	Time for 10 cycles: 40–53 sec.		
5. Call for Switch	Compressor calls for switch when fatigued.	Give clear signal to change.		
		Compressor completes 5th compression.		
		Ventilator completes ventilation after 5th compression.		
6. Switch	Simultaneously switch:			
	Ventilator moves to chest.	Move to chest.		
		Become compressor.		
		Get into position for compressions.		
		Locate landmark notch.		
	Compressor moves to head.	Move to head.		
		Become ventilator.		
		Check carotid pulse (5 sec).		
		Say "No pulse."		
		Ventilate once.†		
7. Continue CPR	Resume compression/ventilation cycles.	Resume Step 4.		

*(a) If CPR is in progress with one rescuer (lay person), the entrance of the two rescuers occurs after the completion of one rescuer's cycle of 15 compressions and 2 ventilations. The EMS should be activated first. The two new rescuers start with Step 6. (b) If CPR is in progress with one professional rescuer, the entrance of a second professional res- cuer is at the end of a cycle after check for pulse by first rescuer. The new cycle starts with one ventilation by the first rescuer, and the second rescuer becomes the compressor.

† During practice and testing only one rescuer actually ventilates the manikin. The other rescuer simulates ventilation.

Instructor _____ Check: Satisfactory _____ Unsatisfactory _____

4/86

CPR and ECC Performance Sheet
Two-Rescuer CPR: Child*

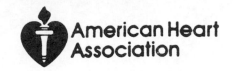
American Heart Association

Name _____ Date _____

Step	Activity	Critical Performance	S	U
1. Airway	One rescuer (ventilator): Assessment: Determines unresponsiveness.	Tap or gently shake shoulder.		
		Shout "Are you OK?"		
	Positions the victim.	Turn on back if necessary (4–10 sec).		
	Opens the airway.	Use a proper technique to open airway.		
2. Breathing	Assessment: Determines breathlessness.	Look, listen and feel (3–5 sec).		
	Ventilator ventilates twice.	Observe chest rise: 1–1.5 sec/inspiration.		
3. Circulation	Assessment: Determines pulselessness.	Feel for carotid pulse (5–10 sec).		
	States assessment results.	Say "No pulse."		
	Other rescuer (compressor): Gets into position for compressions.	Hands, shoulders in correct position.		
	Locates landmark notch.	Landmark check.		
4. Compression/Ventilation Cycles	Compressor begins chest compressions.	Correct ratio compressions/ventilations: 5/1.		
		Compression rate: 80–100/min (5 compressions/3–4 sec).		
		Say any helpful mnemonic.		
		Stop compressing for each ventilation.		
	Ventilator ventilates after every 5th compression and checks compression effectiveness.	Ventilate 1 time (1–1.5 sec/inspiration).		
		Occasionaly palpate pulse to assess compressions.		
	(Minimum of 10 cycles.)	Time for 10 cycles: 40–53 sec.		
5. Call for Switch	Compressor calls for switch when fatigued.	Give clear signal to change.		
		Compressor completes 5th compression.		
		Ventilator completes ventilation after 5th compression.		
6. Switch	Simultaneously switch:			
	Ventilator moves to chest.	Move to chest.		
		Become compressor.		
		Get into position for compressions.		
		Locate landmark notch.		
	Compressor moves to head.	Move to head.		
		Become ventilator.		
		Feel for carotid pulse (5 sec).		
		Say "No pulse."		
		Ventilate once.†		
7. Continue CPR	Resume compression/ ventilation cycles.	Resume Step 4.		

* (a) If CPR is in progress with one rescuer (lay person), the entrance of the two rescuers occurs after the completion of one rescuer's cycle of 5 compressions and 1 ventilation. The EMS should be activated first. The two new rescuers start with Step 6. (b) If CPR is in progress with one professional rescuer, the entrance of a second professional res- cuer is at the end of a cycle after check for pulse by first rescuer. The new cycle starts with one ventilation by the first rescuer, and the second rescuer becomes the compressor.

† During practice and testing only one rescuer actually ventilates the manikin. The other rescuer simulates ventilation.

Instructor _____ Check: Satisfactory _____ Unsatisfactory _____

4/86

Chapter Four

Wounds, Bleeding and Shock

Wounds, especially those that bleed severely, can be very frightening injuries. Because of the bleeding, wounds may cause strong emotional reactions from the injured as well as by-standers. Wounds and hemorrhage (severe bleeding) are both potentially dangerous injuries. Wounds may become infected and may result in such fluid volume loss that the victim may go into shock. *Shock* can be more dangerous than hemorrhaging wounds. Shock is a deadly, quiet killer.

In this chapter, we will discuss types of wounds and shock, hemorrhage associated with various types of wounds, and management of these situations.

Wounds are of two basic types, either **open** or **closed**. Both types of wounds are dangerous, each for a different set of reasons.

OPEN WOUNDS

An *open wound* is one in which the skin has been broken. As a general rule, open wounds are accompanied by some degree of bleeding. Two major considerations must be kept in mind. First, we must determine if bleeding is associated with the open wound and, if it is, we must determine its severity. Secondly, it is important to remember the function of the skin in warding off infections. Any open wound must be carefully monitored to minimize the risk of infection that rises when the skin is broken and the underlying tissues are exposed to the air.

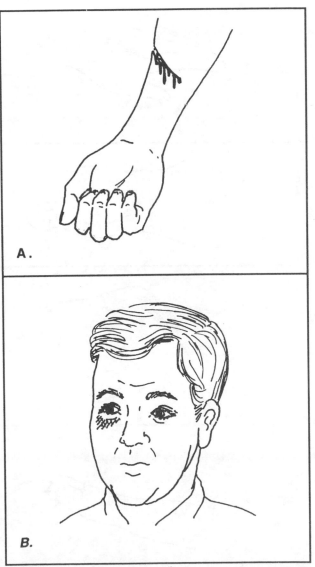

A.

B.

Figure 4-1. *A, open wounds bleed. B, closed wounds don't bleed outside the body. (A black eye is a closed wound.)*

Figure 4-2. *Open wounds are classified into five different categories: incisions, lacerations, punctures, abrasions and avulsions.*

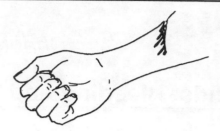

Incised Wounds: These are wounds resulting from a sharp-edged cutting instrument such as a scalpel used in surgery, a razor blade, or a knife. Generally, we think of incisions as occurring from surgery.

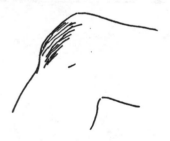

Lacerated Wounds: Lacerated wounds result from a tearing of the skin. Wounds resulting from a tearing of the skin result in jagged edge wounds. Such wounds commonly occur as a result of trauma-related accidents. The jagged edges of these wounds make them more susceptible to infection than incisions.

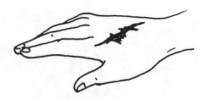

Puncture Wounds: These are wounds which result from a smaller diameter instrument such as an ice pick or nail . These wounds are dangerous because they carry with them a high risk of infection.

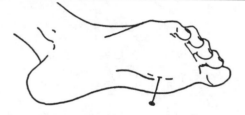

Abrasions: These are wounds which result from a scraping away of the skin, such as in a "floor burn." These wounds are very susceptible to infection and may be very uncomfortable depending on the size and location, but otherwise are not usually dangerous.

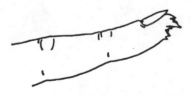

Avulsions: In cases where the skin has been torn loose but not separated from the body, the wound is said to be avulsed. Mechanical equipment and industrial accidents have the potential for pinching and tearing away skin leaving flaps of tissue partially attached. Avulsions are highly susceptible to infection.

CLOSED WOUNDS

Any wound that results in tissue damage but does not cause an opening in the skin is a *closed wound*. Open wounds may hemorrhage externally with loss of blood that may create a life-threatening situation. Closed wounds may create a situation less easily diagnosed, yet equally dangerous.

Any situation with the potential for causing internal damage should be carefully monitored. Among such situations are automobile crashes where the occupants of the vehicles come into contact with interior parts of the car. Especially if not wearing seat belts, passengers may be thrown against gearshift levers, windshields, mirrors, steering wheels, arm rests and any other protrusions in the passenger compartment.

The real danger of undiagnosed internal or closed wounds is that the individual's condition may progressively deteriorate without obvious external signs. A closed wound which begins as minor may progress to a life-threatening situation if not detected. The problem, then, is recognizing internal injuries early. Some injuries require only rest and heat or cold therapy while others require immediate transport to a medical facility. Knowing the difference between a deep bruise and internal hemorrhage may save a life.

Assessment of Closed Wounds

Closed wounds can be difficult to evaluate. Closed wounds are generally assumed from the sum of assessment of the environment in which the victim was injured and the collection of signs and symptoms. Any situation which may have caused blunt trauma (sudden impact to the body) should be suspected of having caused an internal injury. A closed wound should be suspected if any of the following signs are noticed alone or in combination:

1. Abdominal muscle tension (not controlled by the victim)
2. Bruised skin
3. Tenderness
4. Coughing up blood
5. Blood in ears or nose
6. Swelling associated with trauma
7. Recent history suggesting blunt trauma

BLEEDING

In the general sense, hemorrhage refers to severe loss of blood. Hemorrhage may be external (the blood actually exits the body through an opening in the skin) or internal (blood loss is within the body but still not available to fill the needs of the body). Hemorrhage is classified according to the source: arterial, venous or capillary.

> Two injuries which result in dangerous wounds should be mentioned here. First, the fractured femur (discussed in Chapter 6) may cause an open or closed wound in the thigh. It does not matter if the wound is open or closed, the fractured femur may cause loss of one and one-half to two liters of blood. This is sufficient blood loss to cause moderate to severe shock. Secondly, a fractured pelvis (also discussed in Chapter 5) may cause extensive internal blood loss and result in life-threatening shock.

TYPES OF BLEEDING

Arterial hemorrhage is blood loss from an artery. It is easily recognizable as the blood is bright red in color and the loss is rapid. Arterial bleeding may also come in spurts that correspond to the heartbeat.

Venous hemorrhage is blood loss from a vein. As compared to arterial bleeding, the blood will be deep red in color (almost purple) and the flow is a more steady stream. While arterial hemorrhage may result in the loss of a larger amount of blood because of higher inter-arterial pressure, venous hemorrhage is also very serious, since 60% of the total blood volume is in the venous side of circulation.

There is also a danger associated with venous hemorrhage that does not have to do with bleeding—*air embolism*. An air embolism occurs when air enters a large vein that has been opened above the heart, especially in the neck. Blood rushing back to the heart creates a sucking action, which draws blood into the vein causing a bubble which can be fatal when the air reaches the heart or the brain.

Capillary bleeding is usually the result of a superficial wound which results in the ooze of blood from capillaries. Capillary bleeding does not usually cause a threat to life because of blood loss, but poses a threat related to infection, as does any open wound.

First Aid for Open Wounds

The treatment for open wounds depends on severity. Superficial wounds can be treated successfully with simple measures, while severe wounds should be seen by a physician. Wounds that should be seen by a physician are characterized as follows:

- Arterial bleeding — bleeding in spurts corresponding to the pulse.

- Destruction of tissue deeper than the skin.

- Destruction of skin tissue in an area where scarring would interfere with function or be disfiguring, as in the hand or face.

- Contamination of the wound with dirt, wood, manure, or other dangerous material.

- Foreign matter in the wound that cannot be removed by washing.

- Any situation in which there is doubt about the outcome if a physician is not consulted.

Principles of Wound Care

Regardless of severity, four basic principles apply to the care of all wounds.

1. Control bleeding without blocking circulation to undamaged tissue. While control of bleeding is of utmost importance, the technique(s) used to accomplish control should not cut off blood supply excessively.

2. Prevent excessive contamination. Infection is a constant threat with all open wounds. Act in ways to keep the wound as clean as possible at all times. If at all possible, the emergency caregiver should wash his/her hands with soap and water before touching a wound.

3. Apply the proper dressing and bandage. Dressings and the bandages that hold them in place act to control bleeding and keep the wound free of contamination.

4. Transport to medical care. In cases where medical attention is critical to survival or to achieving a good outcome, transport should be a high priority.

Triage. When there are two or more injured people requiring emergency care, decisions about which victim should be treated first must be made quickly. Triage is the term that describes the process of evaluating victims and assigning priority for emergency care. Severe injuries and life threatening conditions should be given care first. Those not breathing and/or without heartbeat require immediate care. Those with severe uncontrolled bleeding or severe burns are the second priority. Victims in shock come next, followed by those with fractures and other injuries. Victims clearly beyond help are the final priority.

METHODS FOR CONTROLLING BLEEDING

Four methods can be used to control bleeding: direct pressure, elevation, pressure points and the tourniquet. The first three methods function very effectively, and will control bleeding in nearly all cases. The tourniquet should only be used when the first three methods fail.

Direct pressure and elevation. Direct pressure and elevation are discussed together because in nearly all cases they should be used together. These two methods will control serious bleeding in all but the most severe cases.

Direct pressure should be applied over the wound, preferably with a sterile dressing under the hand. If a sterile dressing is unavailable, any clean

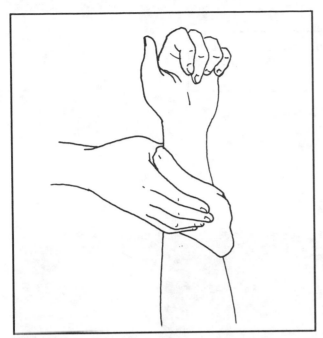

Figure 4-3. *Direct pressure and elevation will control bleeding in most cases.*

piece of cloth will suffice. Do not use absorbent cotton or any material that will come apart if it becomes soaked with blood, for it may become imbedded in the wound.

Use only enough pressure to control the bleeding. Too much pressure may interrupt circulation to other parts of the body or cause further damage. Depending on the location of the wound, light pressure may be enough. Deep wounds on fleshy parts of the body (the upper thigh, for example) will require more pressure.

Elevate the wound above the level of the heart, if possible. This procedure will use gravity to aid in controlling bleeding and may help ease pain. Use common sense in applying direct pressure and elevation to control bleeding. Do not apply pressure or elevation when the actions could cause further injury.

In general, great care should be exercised in using direct pressure and elevation for wounds that are associated with fractures. Elevation should not be attempted until a proper splint has been applied, and direct pressure should not be used over a fracture.

Pressure Points. There are several locations in the human body where arteries pass between the surface and bone. Pressure on the surface at these locations blocks the blood supply. These locations are known as "pressure points" and are extremely useful for controlling bleeding in cases where direct pressure and elevation are not effective or cannot be used safely. Figure 4-5 shows the location of the pressure points most useful in controlling bleeding.

In using pressure points, two important objectives for control of bleeding are achieved: the amount of blood reaching the wound is reduced and the clotting mechanisms of the body can begin to control the bleeding "naturally." In using pressure points, it is important that the tips of the fingers *not* be used—use the fingers. Do not use pressure points any longer than necessary. For severe bleeding where direct pressure and elevation cannot be used, use a pressure point to control bleeding long enough to inspect the wound and apply a bulky dressing and bandage. Release the pressure as soon as possible.

Tourniquet. The tourniquet is the last resort, and should only be used when bleeding cannot be controlled by any of the other methods. When deciding to use this method, consider probable loss of the limb below the tourniquet as the cost, saving a life as the benefit. Loss of the limb is likely because when the blood supply is cut off, the tissues below the tourniquet will probably die. Regardless, if bleeding is such that it cannot be controlled with direct pressure, elevation, and pressure points, the tourniquet must be used.

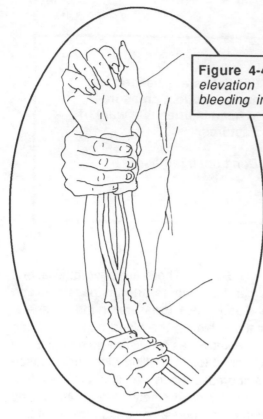

Figure 4-4. Combining direct pressure, elevation and pressure points will control bleeding in most cases.

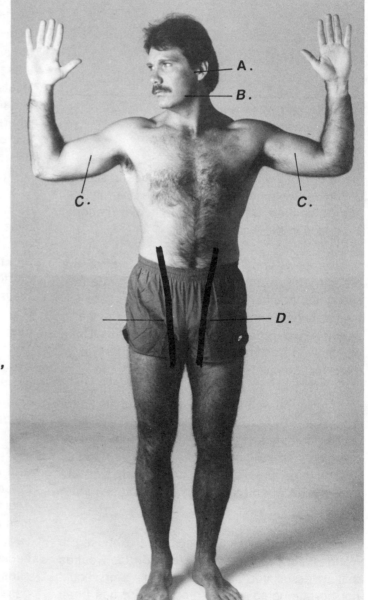

Figure 4-5. Pressure points: A, temporal; B, facial; C, brachial; D, femoral.

82

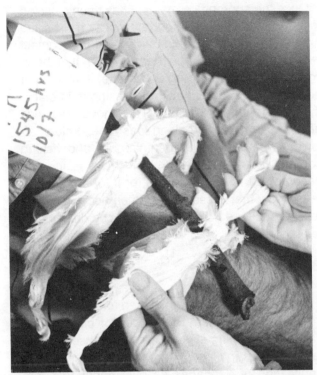

Figure 4-6. *Apply the tourniquet as a last resort to control bleeding. Hold the stick (used to twist the cravat) in place with a second triangular bandage. Never cover a tourniquet and be sure to note the time applied and the date.*

In using the tourniquet:

— Tighten only enough to control the bleeding (see Figure 4-6).

— Once the tourniquet is applied, never loosen or remove.

— Always indicate the time applied, using a prominent tag on the victim. (Write on the forehead with lipstick, for example.)

— To help make certain it is noticed, never cover the tourniquet. (Victims with tourniquets receive priority care in triage.)

— Remain with the victim until you are relieved and communicate needed information about the tourniquet.

— If bleeding persists without control, add another tourniquet without removing the first.

First Aid for Superficial Wounds

A superficial wound is one that involves minimal tissue destruction. Bleeding is controlled easily, requiring use of pressure points only in rare circumstances. The first aid for such wounds is also simple:

1. Wash your hands with soap and water.

2. Cleanse the wound with soap and water, controlling bleeding with gentle, direct pressure.

3. Apply a dressing and bandage.

Soap and water work best for treatment of superficial wounds. There is no need for disinfectants or ointments.

Wounds and Tetanus

Open wounds, particularly puncture wounds, place the victim at risk for a variety of infections. Tetanus is one of the more important infections, given the severe effects it can produce. The question of tetanus should be addressed for all puncture wounds in particular, and all open wounds in general. *Tetanus* can be prevented by a long-lasting immunization or by injection of antibodies for those exposed to the disease in the unprotected state. Ask all victims with open wounds when they received their tetanus shot. If they cannot remember or if it was at least five years ago, they should consult a physician about a booster.

First Aid for Closed Wounds

As for open wounds, first aid for closed wounds differs according to the apparent seriousness of the wound. Keeping in mind the fact that closed wounds are more difficult to assess than open wounds because surface damage is limited, first aid consists of two essential procedures: apply cold and transport to medical facilities for prompt treatment.

For closed wounds judged to be serious, keep the victim quiet and transport to a medical facility. Victims may experience severe pain and thirst, may not be able to find a position that is comfortable, or may become nauseated. Do not give the victim anything to eat or drink, since surgery may be necessary and food or drink can complicate anesthesia. Shock is an important indication that a closed wound is serious.

For superficial closed wounds (a black eye without damage to the eye itself, for example), application of cold—a cold, wet compress and not a steak!—will help to stop the internal bleeding and minimize the bruising.

DRESSING AND BANDAGING WOUNDS

The second phase of hemorrhage treatment is dressing and bandaging the wound. During this phase of treatment it is very important to clean the area and keep it as clean as possible. The wound must be protected from exposure to environmental contaminants and care must be taken to avoid introducing contamination as a part of treatment. Maintaining a clean environment around the wound is not a separate procedure which takes precedence over hemorrhage control, but rather is a process followed as first aid progresses and is meant to minimize contamination of the wound and surrounding area. We must do these things as we go about the second part of hemorrhage control.

Dressings

Dressings are nothing more than sterile coverings for open wounds. If sterile commercial dressings are not available, the rescuer should use the cleanest material available. The chosen dressing must be of sufficient size to cover the wound completely. Dressings should not be improvised from material made of cloth that will come apart if wet, since the material may become imbedded in the wound and create subsequent problems.

Once the appropriate material has been selected for the dressing, it is important not to handle the area of the dressing which will come into contact with the wound. Once hemorrhage has been controlled and a dressing is in place, it should not be removed. Soon after the dressing is in place, the clotting process begins. To remove dressings after this is to risk breaking loose these clots, allowing hemorrhage to begin again and risking contamination to the wound. If the dressing has become saturated with blood, or if for some other reason another dressing becomes necessary, the rescuer must add dressings to existing dressings.

Bandages

A bandage is any material used to secure dressings. Bandages may be pieces of cloth, belts, gauze, or anything else which can be used to fasten dressings in place. Care must be taken in the application of bandages as over-eager rescuers sometimes tie bandages too tightly and restrict blood supply to the affected area. Bandages must be tight enough to secure the dressing, but not so tight as to become a tourniquet or constricting band. The most effective and easy-to-use bandage is a self-adherent roller bandage. The self-adhering bandage conforms to irregular surfaces and may be used by the inexperienced rescuer without a great deal of training. Once the bandage has been applied, be sure there are no loose ends of the bandaging or dressing material. Tuck or tie loose ends out of the way.

AIDS and Open Wounds: Protect Yourself
Blood from another individual may potentially transmit certain diseases, such as AIDS and, most commonly, hepatitis B. Therefore, you should attempt to avoid having a patient's blood come in contact with an open cut or break in your skin. All blood should immediately be washed from your skin after contact to insure minimal risk of disease transmission. If possible, always use gloves when bleeding wounds are involved. Professional care-givers use gloves routinely.

MATERIALS AND METHODS FOR BANDAGING

Although there is an increasing variety of first aid supplies available, all competent emergency care-givers need to be able to fashion dressings and bandages out of commonly available materials. Injuries often occur in situations where "high tech" materials are not available (or don't work!). The basic materials needed for bandaging are triangular bandages (plain cotton cloth 55 inches across the base, 36 to 44 inches on the sides), two--inch roller gauze or its equivalent, and dressing material (see Figure 4-7). These simple materials can be used to bandage a surprisingly wide variety of injuries. Additional materials that make the job of bandaging easier include bandaids, butterfly bandages and adhesive tape.

To prevent additional contamination, it is always best to use sterile dressings on an open wound. Dressings can be purchased in prepackaged sterile wrappers. Open the wrapper carefully to avoid contaminating the dressing—don't touch the dressing (see Figure 4-8). If sterile dressings are not available, use the cleanest material available for

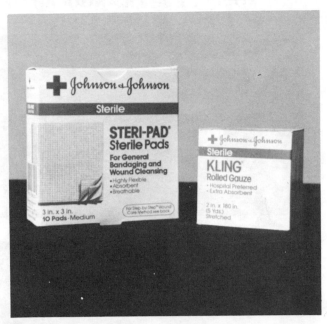

Figure 4-7. *Bandaging materials.*

the dressing. Select materials that will not come apart if soaked with blood or water, such as absorbent cotton. The pieces can stick to the wound and cause a lot of discomfort when removed. Remember: *Dressings are for wounds; bandages are to hold the dressing in place.*

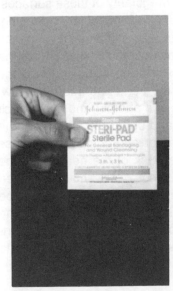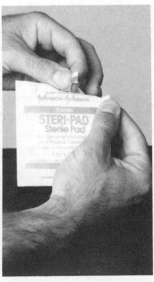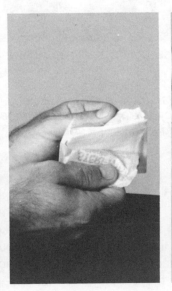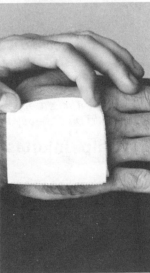

Figure 4-8. *Opening and applying a sterile dressing.*

FOLDING A TRIANGULAR BANDAGE INTO A CRAVAT

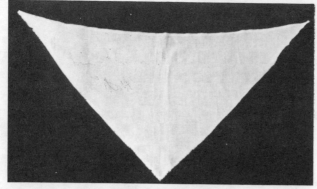

1. Lay out the triangular bandage

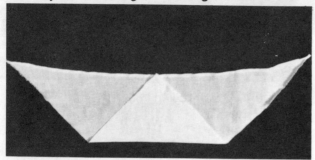

2. Fold peak to base

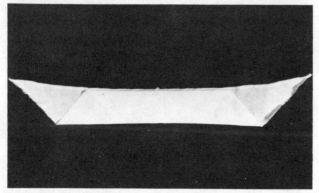

3. Fold peak to base again; continue until 2-3 inches wide.

Figure 4-9. *Triangular bandages are extremely useful for emergency care. These bandages should be carefully folded to form a cravat.*

Scalp Injuries

To bandage a scalp injury, begin with a dressing placed directly over the wound. To hold the dressing in place, use a triangular bandage. Make a hem on the base of the triangular bandage about 2 inches wide and place the bandage on the victim's head. Arrange the bandage so the hem is just above the eyebrows. Wrap the tails of the triangular bandage around the head, keeping the apex of the triangle next to the scalp. Tie the ends off over the forehead using a square knot. Tug on the apex of the triangle to put slight pressure on the dressing and fold as shown in Figure 4-10. If the wound is bleeding severely and the dressing becomes soaked, remove the triangular bandage and add more dressings. Do not remove the soaked dressings. Replace the triangular bandage.

Forehead and Eyes

Wounds to the forehead or the tissues around the eyes require a dressing and a triangular bandage folded into a cravat. Place the dressing on the wound, place the middle of the triangular bandage over the dressing and wrap the tails around the head. Secure the bandage with a square knot over the wound if pressure is needed to control bleeding. Cover both eyes if the tissues around the eyes are involved. If an injury to the eye itself occurs, place a cup or other spacing device over the affected eye to prevent pressure on the injured eye. Remember, additional emotional support, guidance and TLC (tender, loving care) are very important to victims who cannot see.

Face, Ear and Jaw

Bandaging the face, ear or jaw present a challenge because of the irregularity of these surfaces. To use the supplies at our disposal for bandaging, begin by folding a triangular bandage into a cravat, after placing a dressing over the wound. Place the middle of the cravat over the dressing and wrap the ends over the top of the head and under the jaw. Fold the ends across one another and come back across the forehead and under the jaw. Fold the ends across one another and come back across the forehead and the back of the head. Tie the ends off with a square knot. Care should be taken in not making the cravat so tight that it cannot be removed easily. Should the victim become nauseated, a common occurrence with head injuries, the bandage would need to be removed to allow the victim to open his or her mouth to vomit.

For large victims, triangular bandages may not be large enough to function well. Tie two together!

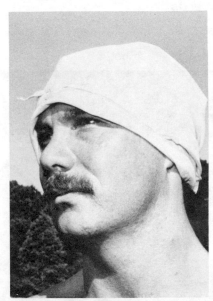

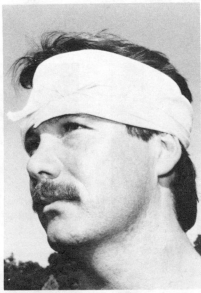

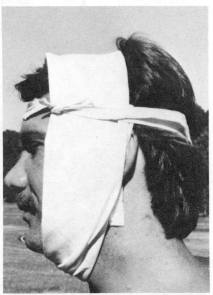

Figure 4-10. *Scalp bandage.* **Figure 4-11.** *Bandage for fore-head and eyes.* **Figure 4-12.** *Bandage for injury to cheek or ear.*

Shoulder

The shoulder area is another irregular surface, like the face and jaw, that requires improvisation for bandaging. Beginning with placement of a dressing, fold two triangular bandages together to make the bandage. Make one into a cravat, folding in the peak of the triangle of the second bandage as you go. Place the cravat near the neck of the victim and tie it off on the front of the chest near the armpit (Fig. 4-13). *Never tie off a bandage over the back of the neck, in the armpit or groin where moving or laying down on the knot can cause discomfort.* Wrap the ends of the second triangular bandage around the upper arm and tie it off to hold the dressing in place. This bandaging technique can also be used for hip injuries.

Chest (sucking chest wounds)

Injuries to the chest can result in open wounds that result in special care. When a chest wound extends through the chest wall, such as might occur with a gunshot wound, the vacuum inside the thorax may be broken. When the vacuum is broken, the injury is called a "sucking chest wound." The broken chest vacuum causes breathing difficulties that may complicate the situation. On encountering a sucking chest wound, the emergency caregiver should immediately try to seal off the wound, taking care not to aggravate the injury. Using a dressing, covered with plastic wrap, foil or other material that can be used to make an airtight seal, cover the wound. Prepare a cravat, two or three if the victim is large, and place around the victim to hold the dressing and seal securely in place. If there is no reason not to (a foreign body in the wound or broken ribs that move), place a magazine or soft cover book over the dressing and tie the cravats over the wound to make a tight seal. It may also help to have the victim exhale before tieing the cravats. If the cravats cause pain, remove them immediately, hold the dressing in place and transport the victim to medical help. *Place the victim on the injured side to help breathing.* See Fig. 4-14.

Figure 4-13. *Bandaging shoulder wounds.*

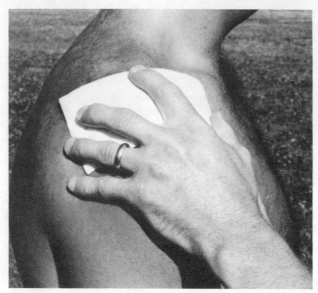

A. *The shoulder is an irregular surface to bandage.*

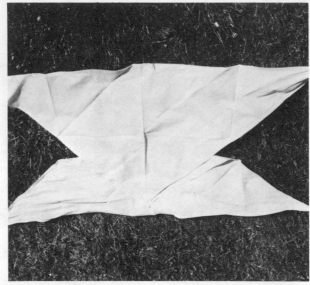

B. *Using two triangular bandages folded together will provide a bandage to hold a dressing over a shoulder injury.*

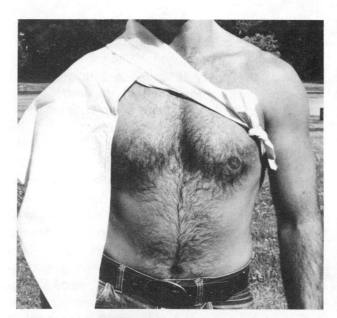

C. *Shoulder bandage.*

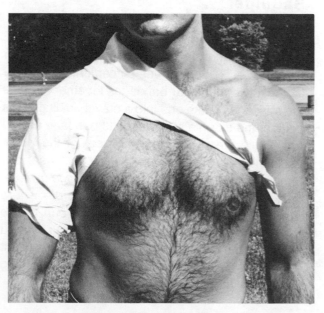

D. *Shoulder bandage completed.*

Figure 4-14. *Bandaging chest wounds.*

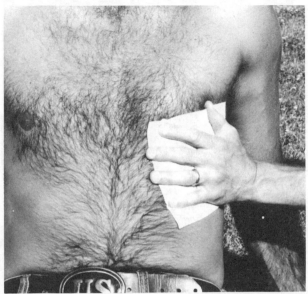

A. For a sucking chest wound, begin with a sterile dressing place directly over the wound and hold it firmly in place.

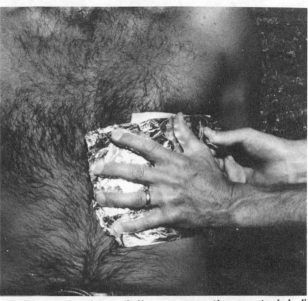

B. Place aluminum foil or some other material directly over the dressing to make an airtight seal.

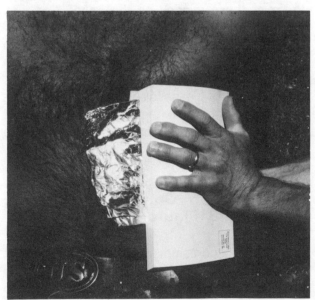

C. Place a book or other firm object over the wound before binding. The solid object will help to apply even pressure on the wound.

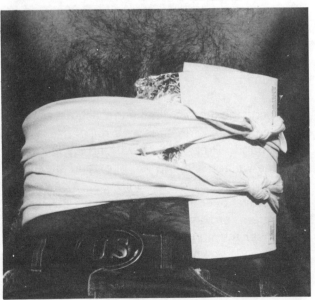

D. As a final step, apply cravats to hold the dressing in place. Have the victim **exhale** as you tighten the cravats. These cravats should be used for large victims or for wounds higher up on the rib cage.

Figure 4-15. *Bandaging palm wounds.*

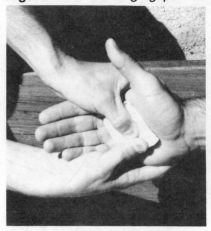 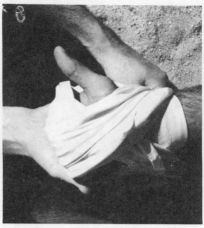 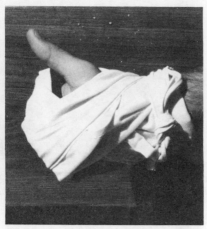

A. Place a large, bulky dressing directly on the wound. Ask the victim to make a fist to help control bleeding.

B. Place the middle of the cravat over the wrist (palm side up) and drape the ends of the cravat over the back of the hand. Now pull the cravat tight over the figures.

C. Tie the cravat off over the wrist, taking care not to make the victim uncomfortable. Leave the thumb exposed to allow for checking circulation.

Palm Pressure

Bandaging lacerations and incision wounds to the palm offers a unique opportunity to the emergency caregiver. Direct pressure can be used to control bleeding by placing a thick dressing (a roll of gauze for example), over the wound and asking the victim to make a fist. A bandage can be fashioned to hold the "fist" in place, the victim can relax the forearm muscles and bleeding control will be maintained.

To bandage the "fist," have the victim make a fist with a bulky dressing such as a roll of gauze in his or her hand. Prepare a cravat and lay the middle over the wrist. Have the victim extend the thumb, to allow circulation to be monitored, cross the ends of the cravat over the back of the wrist and up over the fingers (proximal to distal). Cross the cravat ends over the fingertip side of the fist, and firmly pull the ends down toward the wrist. Tie the cravat off on the wrist. Look at the thumb and check its color. If the thumb is a different color from the thumb on the uninjured hand, the bandage may be too tight.

Bag Bandages

For injuries such as abrasions and mild burns, a light bandage may be needed to keep dirt out of a wound. The triangular bandage can easily be used to cover these injuries on the hands and feet. These bandages can be called "bag bandages" because they resemble a bag placed over the hand or foot. Begin by placing the hand or foot in the middle of a fully extended triangular bandage. Fold the peak of the triangle toward the wrist or ankle and wrap the peak of the triangle toward the wrist or ankle and wrap the ends of the bandage around same to hold the "bag" in place (Fig. 4-16).

Working with Gauze: Anchoring, Spirals and Figure Eights

Gauze is used commonly for bandaging limbs. Used properly, gauze has the advantages of being adaptable to a wide range of wounds, can be used on "tapered" limbs without slipping, and can be applied so as not to be bulky.

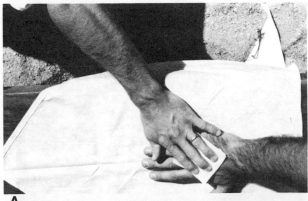

A.

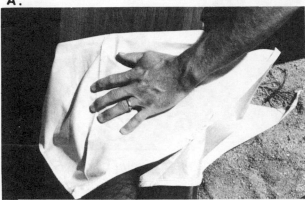

B.

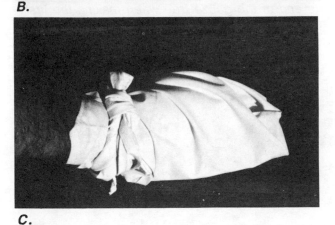

C.

Anchoring the Gauze. To begin, anchor the gauze to hold it in place before covering the dressing. Leaving 1-2 inches free, make one revolution around the limb. Now fold the free end over the gauze on the limb and make another revolution. This will hold the gauze in place. Anchoring works better if applied at non—tapered places such as the wrist or ankle (Fig. 4-17).

Open and Closed Spirals. For tapered limbs such as forearms and lower legs, spiral bandages function well. The gauze will not slip if the bandage is properly applied.

An open spiral should resemble a barber pole. After anchoring, wrap the gauze up the limb leaving gaps between each revolution. This bandage will hold a dressing in place while allowing for some air circulation to the wound. Abrasions, healing wounds, and other situations where primary need for the bandage is to hold the dressing in place are well suited for use of the open spiral.

The closed spiral bandage is useful for situations where the wound needs a tighter bandage than can be provided by an open spiral. Beginning with an anchor, wrap the gauze around the limb, with each revolution covering about one third of the width of the gauze on the limb. To provide greater coverage the procedure can be continued without interruption at the end of the bandage by reversal. A reversing spiral is produced by rotating the gauze 180 degrees proceeding to wrap in the opposite direction, covering the gauze on the limb. Reversing prevents gaps in the gauze from developing and maintains a tight bandage (Fig. 4-18).

Figure 4-16. *Bag bandages help keep superficial wounds clean.*

A. Lay the hand (or foot) in the middle of a triangular bandage.

B. Fold the point of the triangle over the hand.

C. Wrap the ends of the triangular bandage around the wrist (or ankle) to secure the bandage.

Figure 4-17. *Anchoring the bandage.*

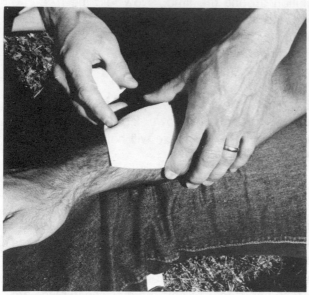

A. *Always place a sterile dressing directly over the wound.*

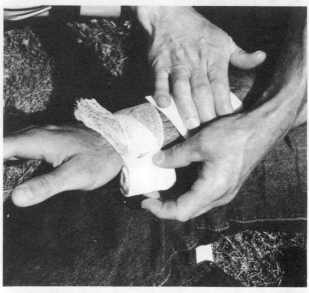

B. *Anchoring holds the gauze in place. For best results, choose a place on the limb that is not tapered to enclose the gauze. Leave 1 - 2 inches of the end of the gauze free when making the first revolution around the limb.*

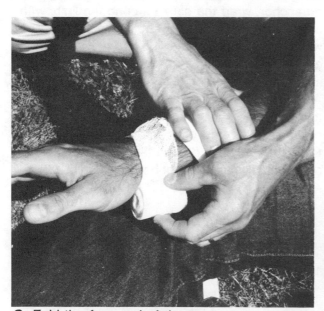

C. *Fold the free end of the gauze over onto the first revolution and rewrap around the limb at least one more time to secure the gauze.*

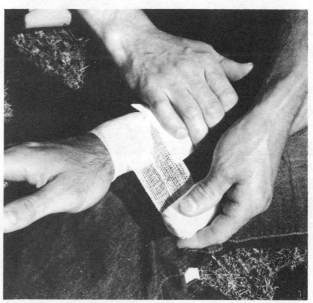

D. *The completed anchor.*

Figure 4-18. *Closed spirals.*

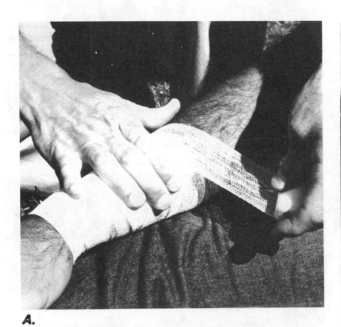

A.

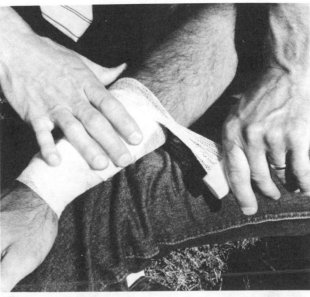

B.

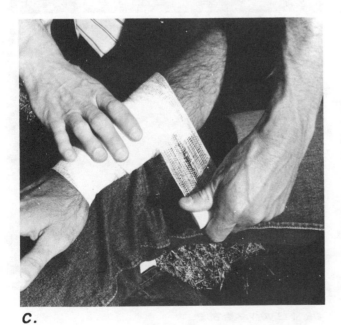

C.

A. The enclosed spiral bandage applies pressure to the sound evenly and keeps dirt out.

B. Rewinding the gauze allows the closed spiral dressing to go up and down the limb, keeping the gauze tight throughout. To reverse rotate the roll of gauze 180 degrees.

C. The completed closed spiral with a reversal at the proximal (elbow) end.

Figure Eight Bandages. Figure eight bandages are well suited to wounds on elbows, knees, and other surfaces that involve motion. Begin by anchoring the gauze and wrap over the

dressing around the limb and back over the dressing. The gauze should make an "X" over the dressing. Tie the gauze off over the anchor.

Figure 4-19. *Figure Eight bandages.*

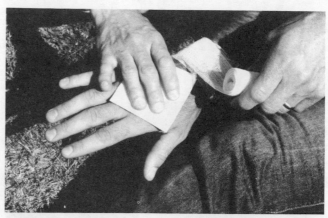

A. Begin as always with a dressing over the wound. Anchor the gauze near the wound.

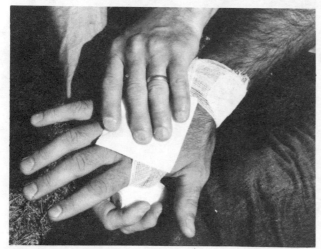

B. Begin the figure eight by crossing the gauze over the dressing.

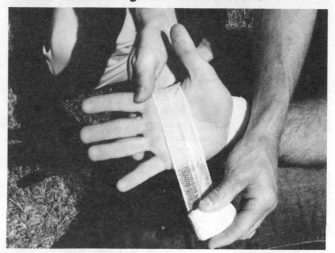

C. Continue wrapping around the injured part.

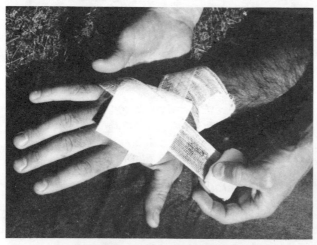

D. Cross the gauze directly over the dressing. The added pressure of the figure eight will help control bleeding while allowing the victim to move the limb without ruining the bandage.

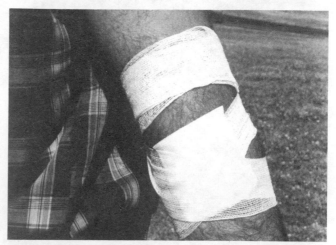

E. A figure eight on the elbow. This type of bandage is very versatile.

Finger and Toe Bandages. Finger and toe wounds have the unfortunate characteristic of developing into throbbing, painful injuries. Any bandage that puts pressure on the wound will make the pain and throbbing worse. The basic rule for these bandages, therefore, is to keep the needs of the victim in mind and ask how tight the bandage should be. Since bleeding is rarely life threatening for lacerated fingers or toes, a relatively loose bandage will probably suffice.

Begin by laying the gauze over itself to form a pad (6-8 inches long for a finger, 4-5 inches long for a toe). Place the middle of the pad over the top of the injured toe(s) or finger(s), drape the gauze down each side, and gently wrap gauze around to hold the pad in place. If throbbing and pain are severe, extend the gauze around the wrist or ankle to avoid having to tie off the gauze near the wound.

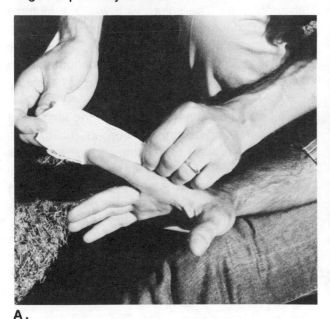

A.

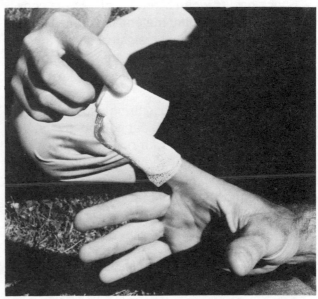

B.

Figure 4-20. *Finger and toe bandages.*

A. Injured fingers and toes need careful attention. A bandage applied too tightly will make throbbing worse. Begin the bandage with a bulky dressing wrapped loosely.

B. Wrap gauze around the injured finger once the dressing is in place.

C. Complete the bandage by tying off at the wrist.

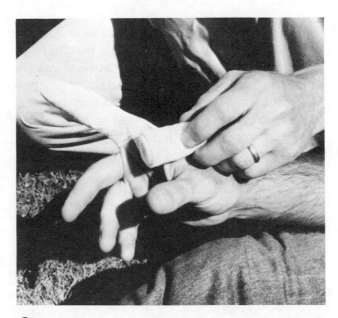

C.

SHOCK

The rest of this chapter is concerned with shock. Shock is a condition that often accompanies serious wounds. It may also develop when no serious injury occurs however. The main objectives for the emergency caregiver, in cases of shock, are to recognize the signs and symptoms early and take steps to prevent shock from deepening.

Shock occurs when blood supply to the body is reduced to the point that basic processes are interrupted. Although the signs of shock are relatively clear, the changes that are occurring in the body as shock develops are very complex.

The importance of recognizing shock early in its course of development cannot be overstated. Many accident victims with nonfatal injuries have died from shock. Consequently, recognizing the signs and providing emergency first aid for shock is one of the most important tasks of the emergency caregiver.

The term *shock* is used to describe several different types of conditions, although all essentially involve lack of adequate blood supply to the body.

TYPES OF SHOCK

Shock Due to Low Volume of Fluids

Hypovolemic shock refers to a loss of enough circulating volume of fluids which in turn compromises the system. The cause of volume depletion may be external loss, as in an open wound, or internal, as in internal hemorrhage. No matter the cause, something must be done to stop the fluid loss if this type of shock is to be controlled.

Metabolic shock is the result of the loss of body fluids over a long period of time (usually) as a result of an untreated disease or illness. Treatment for this type of shock *requires the replacement of fluids by intravenous route; therefore, acquiring medical attention is of the utmost importance.*

Shock Due to Dilated Vessels

This type of shock is the result of an exaggerated allergic reaction to something introduced into the body. The substance introduced may be the poison of an insect sting or ingestion of some food or medicine which proves to be an allergen.

Anaphylactic shock causes the victim to itch, have a headache and eventually develop breathing problems. The speed with which symptoms develop is dependent on the severity of the reaction to the allergen. In some cases, the reaction may develop over a period of several hours and in some cases it may develop in a matter of minutes.

If the reaction is severe enough, the vessels of the throat may become engorged (filled) with blood and suffocate the victim. If the reaction is severe and you are not near medical help an injection of antihistamine and epinephrine may be administered if the victim has an anti-allergenic kit. If no antitoxin is available and the reaction is severe, all you can do is to keep the victim in a position that will ease breathing efforts. Stay ready to administer artificial respiration and transport the victim to the nearest medical facility.

Neurogenic Shock. This situation arises when an injury to the nervous system causes the vessels to dilate, thus reducing venous return and causing shock. Little can be done outside of general treatment and seeking medical attention.

Septic Shock. This type of shock results from a bacterial infection which is then carried via the blood to various sites in the body. The bacteria responsible for the infection release endotoxins which cause blood vessels to dilate and blood to pool. The end result is sharp drop in blood pressure resulting in shock. This type of shock is commonly referred to as blood poisoning.

Psychogenic Shock. This condition results from a sudden overwhelming sensitization of the central nervous system which causes dilation of vessels terminating in fainting. This condition may also result from remaining in the same position motionless for a long period of time. This inactivity causes a loss of the massaging action of the muscles on the vessels returning to the heart. The result is dilation of the vessels and a decrease of returning venous flow followed by fainting.

Shock Due to Pump Failure

Cardiogenic Shock. Cardiogenic shock is a result of the inability of the heart to maintain blood supply to the body. As a general rule, cardiogenic shock is the result of heart disease or acute myocardial infarction. One can only seek medical attention and stand ready to administer cardiopulmonary resuscitation.

Respiratory Shock. Respiratory shock comes about when there is insufficient oxygen in the blood to maintain vital functions. If such a condition persists, the body begins to suffer low oxygen levels. The lungs can be affected and a condition known as **shock lung** results. The kidneys may shut down in an attempt to save fluids causing a dangerous build-up of waste in the blood. Eventually the cardiovascular system and breathing centers may be compromised and shock results. This condition requires immediate medical attention.

PHYSIOLOGY OF SHOCK

If shock is caused by an inadequate blood supply, then it stands to reason that anything which reduces cardiac output can cause shock. The causes of shock may be grouped into three broad categories:

1. Those situations which affect the volume of fluids available in circulation (hypovolemia). An example would be hemorrhage.

2. Those conditions which result in reduced pressure within the cardiovascular network (hypotension) or pumping strength of the heart.

3. **Those situations which result in the loss of control of vasoconstriction and vasodilation** (narrowing and widening of the vessels).

An example would be injury to the spinal cord resulting in loss of nervous control of the muscular walls of the vessels.

Shock Cycle

Shock can be divided into three categories:

1. Nonprogressive stage shock — Blood supply is down but not enough to cause shock to progress.

2. Progressive stage shock — Blood supply is now so deficient that the cardiovascular system is deteriorating. The body cannot reverse this situation and the person will move on to the third type of shock without intervention.

3. Irreversible stage shock — No matter what is done, the person will die from shock even with the return of cardiac function and arterial pressure.

As an example of the cyclic nature of progressive and irreversible stage shock let us look at an example of a severely hemorrhaging wound and the progressive stage shock which may result.

1. Blood volume loss externally (less blood coming back to the heart so the heart pumps faster.)

2. Drop in arterial pressure (special nerve centers [*baroreceptors*] sense this and send messages to the heart.)

3. Heart rate increases (as result of what happened in #1 and #2.)

4. Constricted vessels in the extremities causes blood to be trapped in the core of the body in an attempt to conserve body heat.

5. Low levels of oxygen in tissue.

6. Decreased oxygenation of the breathing centers causing rapid shallow breathing.

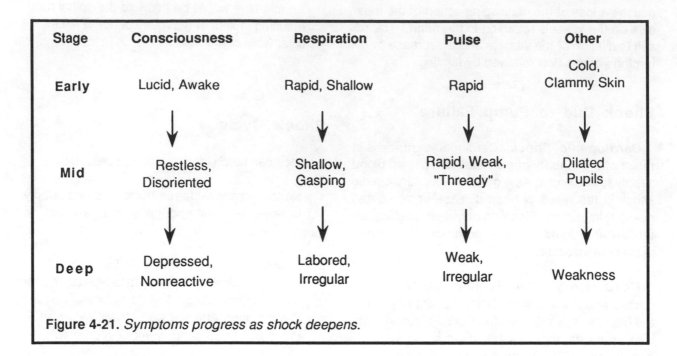

Stage	Consciousness	Respiration	Pulse	Other
Early	Lucid, Awake	Rapid, Shallow	Rapid	Cold, Clammy Skin
	↓	↓	↓	↓
Mid	Restless, Disoriented	Shallow, Gasping	Rapid, Weak, "Thready"	Dilated Pupils
	↓	↓	↓	↓
Deep	Depressed, Nonreactive	Labored, Irregular	Weak, Irregular	Weakness

Figure 4-21. *Symptoms progress as shock deepens.*

7. Loss of fluids through weakened capillaries (increasing loss of fluid to the system.)

8. Pooling of blood in large vessels of the gut.

Classic Symptoms of Shock

Understanding the progressive nature of what happens physiologically in the process, it is easy to relate the symptoms of shock to what is going on in the body. As the classic symptoms are discussed, refer to the previous section and the discussion of the shock cycle. Depending on the stage of shock and the degree of deterioration of the cardiovascular system, you may find some of all of the following symptoms:

1. The skin will be of ashen or grey color and the quality will be clammy (cool, moist and sticky.)

2. The heart rate will be fast and the quality will be thready (rapid, regular but faint or weak.)

3. The blood pressure will be below normal and deteriorate over time.

4. Restlessness, anxiety, and thirst.

In later stages as oxygen deficit affects the brain these additional symptoms will be present:

5. Breathing becomes rapid and shallow.

6. Pupils become dilated because of the de-oxygenation of the breathing centers of the brain.

7. Patient becomes lethargic and complacent followed by stupor and coma.

8. Death will occur without aggressive first aid followed by medical care.

FIRST AID

Just as there are general symptoms for shock, there are some guidelines for treatment which are applicable to all forms of shock. Remember the three broad categories for factors which cause shock: things which cause insufficiency of blood, insufficient blood pressure, and body reactions that reduce venous return of blood.

The immediate priorities in treating shock are:

— insure respiration

— insure heartbeat

— control bleeding

After dealing with the immediate life-threatening injuries, you should take care of fractures. Immobilize all fractures before you go on. Immobilizing fractures will help to control bleeding and will also alleviate pain. Both of these are contributors to deepening shock.

After hemorrhage and fractures are taken care of the feet should be elevated 8-12 inches to aid in venous return (if the patient is conscious and other injuries do not eliminate this option). If the patient has fractures of the legs and/or spine, elevate the foot-end of the backboard. If the patient is unconscious, protect against airway blockage. If in doubt about elevating feet and legs, leave the victim flat. Another means of aiding venous return is to stop loss of heat from the body of the victim. In this way, constriction of external vessels is controlled and more blood is available. Remember, only controlling loss of body heat; do not automatically add heat to the victim.

Always monitor to be certain that the victim is adequately oxygenated. Low levels of oxygen hasten the cycle of shock.

Finally, constantly monitor the victim's pulse and breathing, even if the victim does not exhibit shock symptoms at first. Any injury that involves hemorrhage, internal injury or a great deal of pain may cause shock to develop. Symptoms may be

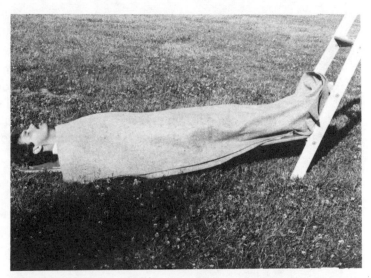

Figure 4-22. *Elevate the feet and legs 8-12 inches to improve circulation for shock victims.*

of rapid onset or they may develop slowly over time. Constant monitoring of pulse, heartbeat, and skin character is imperative with victims of trauma.

****

Remember:

1. Shock is cyclic, and if not reversed, can become life-threatening.

2. The speed with which one acts to intervene in the shock cycle is crucial.

3. Shock can many times become more dangerous than the situation which caused it.

4. Someone with minimal training and no equipment can slow the shock cycle until better-trained and equipped help arrives.

Building Skills: Wounds and Bleeding

There are two separate sets of skill building exercises for this chapter. For wounds and bleeding, the skills are performance of maneuvers needed to control bleeding and apply dressings and bandages. Controlling bleeding and applying appropriate bandages are frequently used first aid skills. To help develop these skills efficiently, review the anatomy section of Chapter 1 before tackling the exercises. Being familiar with the anatomy, particularly circulation of blood, will help you to locate pressure points.

Name_____

Directions:

I. Controlling Bleeding

Satisfactory   Recheck

a. Direct pressure

Demonstrate the correct application
of direct pressure to control bleeding.   _____ _____

b. Pressure points

Find the pulses associated with the following pressure points. Gentle pressure on the pulses should produce mild tingling distal to the pressure. Do not press hard and do not hold for more than 15 seconds.

a. *Facial artery*

Feel for a groove in the bottom of the jawbone
(mandible) about 2/3 of the way toward
the ear   _____ _____

b. *Temporal artery*

Place your index finger on your face directly
in front of your ear to find this pulse.   _____ _____

c. *Brachial artery*

Feel between the biceps and triceps on the
inner surface of the upper arm (relax the
muscles of the arm).   _____ _____

d. *Femoral artery*

Imagine an equilateral triangle about six inches
on each side with the apex on the navel.Feel
for the femoral pulse on the feet of the triangle. _____ _____

e. *Popliteal artery*

Feel directly behind the knee.   _____ _____

c. Tourniquet

Apply a tourniquet on a simulated victim. Assume that this victim has an injury to the left forearm. Direct pressure and elevation have failed to control bleeding. Do not tighten the tourniquet!

a. Correct materials selected   _____ _____
b. Correct techniques used   _____ _____
c. Label used correctly   _____ _____
d. Does not cover   _____ _____

II. Bandages. Simulate appropriate first aid procedures for the injuries listed below. For each injury, apply the correct dressing and bandage and specify how bleeding would best be controlled.

	Satisfactory	Recheck
a. Bleeding laceration on the top of the head		
Scalp dressing	_____	_____
Scalp bandage	_____	_____
Bleeding controlled by	_____	_____
b. Laceration over right eye		
Bleeding heavily	_____	_____
Dressing	_____	_____
Cravat bandage	_____	_____
Bleeding controlled by	_____	_____
c. Laceration on bridge of nose, probably requiring sutures		
Dressing	_____	_____
Cravat bandage over both eyes	_____	_____
Bleeding controlled by	_____	_____
d. Avulsion of part of left outer ear		
Dressing	_____	_____
Cheek/ear cravat bandage	_____	_____
Bleeding controlled by	_____	_____
e. Closed wound of left jaw		
Application of cold	_____	_____
f. Abrasions on left and right elbows		
Dressing	_____	_____
Figure 8 bandages	_____	_____
Bleeding controlled by	_____	_____

g. Severe laceration on left forearm

Dressing   _____   _____

Close spiral with anchor, reversal   _____   _____

Bleeding controlled by   _____   _____

h. Puncture wounds on back of right hand
with heavy bleeding

Dressing   _____   _____

Figure 8 bandage   _____   _____

Bleeding controlled by   _____   _____

　　　　　　　　　Name_____

Directions: You will need to work with at least one partner to complete these exercises. Groups of three are ideal. The goals of the exercises are to explore how assessment of respiration, heartbeat, consciousness and skin reflect changes in the condition of the body.

I. Assessment at rest. Select one member of the group to act as the "victim" for this exercise. This individual should lie down for at least three minutes, not interact with any other people and ideally not become distracted by any other environmental stimuli such as loud noises, etc. When the three minutes have elapsed, carry out and record the measurements listed below.

a. Respiration. Observe the "victim's " chest rise and fall. Place your hand on his chest to help detect breathing if necessary.

rate per minute　　　　_____

regularity: regular　　　_____

　　　　　　variable　　　_____

　　　　　　gasping　　　_____

depth of inhalation:　shallow　_____

　　　　　　　　　　　medium　_____

　　　　　　　　　　　deep　　_____

b. Heartbeat. Measure heart rate using the carotid pulse. Do not reach across the throat.

rate per minute:　　_____

strength of pulse:　strong, distinct　　　_____

　　　　　　　　　　clearly felt but not strong _____

　　　　　　　　　　weak and faint　　　　_____

c. Consciousness. Ask the victim a series of questions to find out the information you need. Ask the victim's name, age, address and other such questions that have clear, unambiguous answers. Avoid questions that require interpretation.

conscious, oriented   _____

disoriented, confused   _____

unconscious   _____

d. Skin character. Observe the victim's skin, looking at color and condition of hair follicles (erect or relaxed). Touch the victim to determine texture. Be sure to include the conditions in the room and their effect on the victim in making judgments.

temperature: cool   _____

     normal   _____

     hot   _____

     chilled, shaking   _____

texture: dry   _____

     normal   _____

     wet   _____

II. Assessment after change. Changes associated with mild exercise simulate changes that might occur in a victim of trauma who was beginning to slip into shock. To carry out this simulation, the "victim" should stand on one leg and jump for 45-60 seconds. All the assessment activities outlined in part one should be repeated.

Respiration:

rate per minute   _____

regularity: regular   _____

     variable   _____

     gasping   _____

depth of inhalation: shallow   _____

     medium   _____

     deep   _____

Name_____

Heartbeat:

rate per minute: _____

strength of pulse: strong, distinct   _____

                         clearly felt but not strong _____

                         weak and faint   _____

Consciousness:

conscious, oriented   _____

disoriented, confused   _____

unconscious   _____

Skin character:

temperature: cool   _____

                 normal   _____

                 hot   _____

                 chilled, shaking   _____

texture: dry   _____

                 normal   _____

                 wet   _____

III. Comparison. Collect the data collected by other member(s) of your group. If there are differences, determine how and why they occurred.

IV. Conclusion. Briefly summarize the data you have collected. How did the data change from Part I to part II?

a. **Respiration** _____

_____

_____

b. **Heartbeat** _____

_____

_____

c. **Consciousness** _____

_____

_____

d. **Skin Character** _____

_____

_____

Chapter Five

Bone and Joint Injuries

The greatest number of bone and joint injuries are recreation-related. Today in our culture, a large percentage of the population engages in physical activities for fun and fitness. With such a large number of people involved in recreational sports, we may expect many injuries as a result of active leisure pursuits. Some people will be injured as a result of the risk involved in these activities while others will be injured as a result of ignorance of proper precautions associated with physical activity, or preventive safety measures.

Many times pain, recuperation time and return to normal function of the limb depends on initially correct handling of the bone or joint. Correct assessment and handling may greatly reduce the possibility of damaging vessels, nerves or other tissues, resulting in a negative outcome from these types of injuries.

Bones

Bones provide several functions. In terms of structural and anatomical functions, they may be divided into three general categories:

1. Bones make motion possible by allowing for a point of attachment for muscle.

2. Bones provide support.

3. Bones protect underlying organs and tissues.

Any time a bone is fractured the resulting loss of these functions must be considered and compensated for.

Bones are divided into four types according to *Gray's Anatomy.* Each type of bone is of a different composition and serves a different purpose. The four types of bones and their purposes are:

Long bones — These are the bones of the extremities, such as the *femur* or *humerus.* They are weight-bearing and are responsible for locomotion.

Short bones — Where the skeleton is compact and strong with little requirement for movement, the short bones are found. These are usually found in groups of small bones held together by ligaments such as the carpals in the hand.

Flat bones — When there is a need to protect large areas as in the bones of the skull, or large muscles need attachment, we find the bones of the skeleton flattened.

Irregular bones — These bones are different to the point that they do not really fit any other classification and hold no similarity with other non-categorized bones.

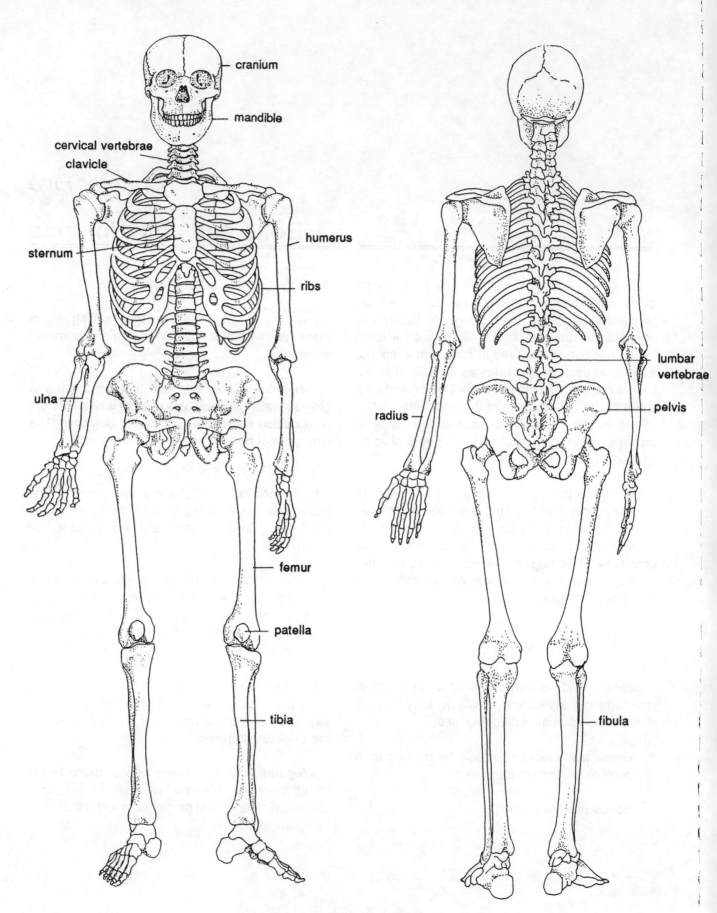

Figure 5-1. *Bones of the body.*

110

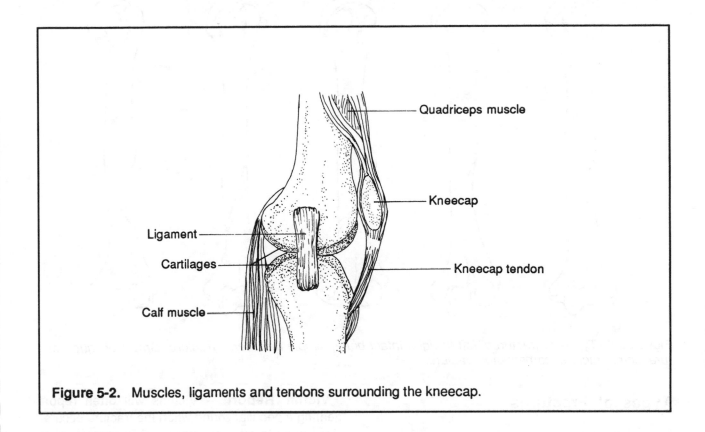

Figure 5-2. Muscles, ligaments and tendons surrounding the kneecap.

MUSCLES, LIGAMENTS, AND TENDONS

Muscles provide the power for motion. To accomplish motion, however, the muscles must be attached to bones on both sides of the movable joints. *Tendons* provide this attachment. In addition, the bones must be attached to one another to provide stability for joints. *Ligaments* attach bone to bone. Each of the movable joints — note that many joints, such as those in the skull, are not movable — consists of a system wherein the bones are joined together in such a way that motion can occur and is powered by muscles.

The injuries to the skeleton and associated structures can be grouped into several categories. These categories include fractures of bones, dislocations of bones in joints, sprains of joints, and strains to muscles.

FRACTURES

Many everyday activities carry with them the potential for accidental injury. In any activity where mechanical energy is transferred, there is the possibility for fractures to occur. In athletics, recreational activities, at work or in automobile accidents, breaks in bones may occur.

In recreation and athletics we see force applied to long bones which are locked in position. Occasionally, force is applied directly to the bone. At work there are falls and crushing injuries which may cause breaks. One of the most common causes of fractures are automobile accidents. Passengers who are not belted in may be thrown about the interior coming into contact with steering wheels, windshields, dashboards, gearshift levers and other accessories in the passenger compartment. Those passengers who are belted in may suffer injuries from lap belts and broken *clavicles* from shoulder harnesses.

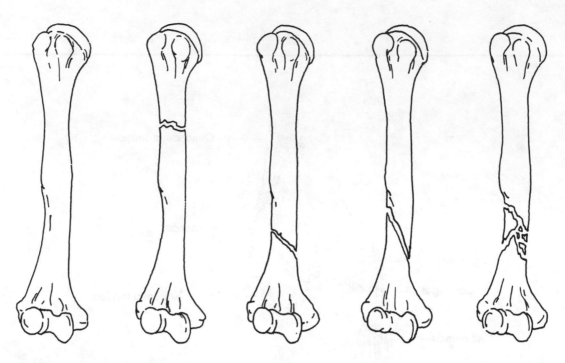

Figure 5-3. *Types of fractures, left to right: Intact bone, simple transverse fracture, simple oblique fracture, spiral fracture, comminuted fracture.*

Types of Fractures

Fractures may be classified as open or closed, simple or complicated. Open fractures occur when there is an open wound associated directly with the fracture. Simple fractures are fractures which occur in the mid shaft of a bone and are considered simple because there is little danger of complication.

More complicated fractures are those in which bones are broken into many fragments, fractures occurring near joints, fractures of the elbow, or those which pose some other risk.

Signs and Symptoms of Fractures

Fractures can only be diagnosed by x-ray, and in many cases what appears to be a fracture turns out to be something else. Of course, when limbs have unusual bends or other deformities, the likelihood of a fracture is high. Therefore, the rule for emergency care givers is to treat all suspected fractures as definite fractures. Fractures are associated with the following.

Victim Report — Victims will often report hearing a peculiar sound when the fracture occurs. The sound is often a "snap" and is accompanied by loss of function in the effected body part.

Crepitus — When fractured bone ends rub together, the sound that is produced is termed "crepitus." This feeling can be described by victims and should alert the emergency care giver to the great possibility of a fracture.

Deformity — Indentations, protrusions and bends in body structures where there should be none are tell-tale signs of deformity. Remember that the body is symmetric, and that corresponding parts — left and right arms, for example — can be compared if there is doubt about a deformity.

Discoloration — Bruising frequently occurs at the site of a fracture because of damage to underlying tissues. Bones also have their own blood supply, and interruption of this supply that occurs with fractures will lead to discoloration.

Swelling — Damage to any body tissue usually results in swelling. In most fractures, swelling will develop shortly after the injury occurs.

Loss of function and pain — Fractures are painful injuries. In many cases, pain will not be apparent until the victim attempts to use the injured body part. Using fractured parts is very painful, and, as swelling progresses, eventually impossible.

Disputing a common myth: A victim may be able to move a limb or body part even if it is fractured.

First Aid for Fractures

The general principles governing emergency care for fractures can be summarized into four key ideas: immobilization, elevation, cold, and "splint 'em as you find 'em."

Immobilization — Support the injured body part and prevent further damage by immobilizing the fracture site. Use the appropriate splint, and in the case of a limb, remember both of the adjacent joints. It is important to include adjacent joints because fractures may be accompanied by muscle spasms which may cause broken bone ends to move against one another and damage the muscles and other tissues in the process.

Elevation — Act to control swelling and reduce pain by elevating the fracture site above the level of the heart *after splinting*.

Cold — Applying cold to a fracture will help control swelling and pain. Do not apply ice directly to the skin.

Splint 'em as you find 'em — Do not move any injured body part unnecessarily. Unless circulation is impaired, as occurs in joint fractures occasionally, the best procedure is to instruct the victim to remain immobile and splint the injured body part in its current position. Movement is likely to cause further injury.

Watch Out for Complications

Remember that fractures are potentially serious injuries. At the very minimum, the presence of a fracture means that the victim suffered sufficient trauma to break a bone. Consequently, shock is a real possibility. When fractures or dislocations occur, the damage to the body may also cause additional injury by blocking nerves and/or arteries.

Always check for feeling and pulse at a point further away from the heart. If the injury has blocked an artery, the victim will not have a pulse below the fracture site. If a nerve has been affected, the victim will feel tingling and/or pain in the limb below the fracture site.

SPLINTS

Splints are nothing more than devices intended to immobilize a bone and adjacent joints. In a fracture the function of support provided by bone is lost, and some artificial means of accomplishing this function must be found. Splinting accomplishes this goal.

Improvised Splints

An improvised splint is exactly what the term implies — a splint that has been constructed from available materials and ingenuity.

The decision to splint is predicated on whether transport or medical help will be available soon. If there is a simple fracture that can be easily splinted and the victim transported to a hospital, then splinting is in order. If the fracture is complicated or medical help will be arriving soon, there is no need to splint. The choice of splinting material should be based on the lightest, easiest to use material. The following is a short listing of types of splints:

Improvised splits (these are splints which are made from materials commonly found at work or home):

A. Pillows
B. Blankets
C. Magazines
D. Boards
E. Books
F. Sling and swathe [This is usually available commercially or may be improvised. It is nothing more than a triangular piece of cloth (sling) and wide strips of cloth used to bind (swathe).]

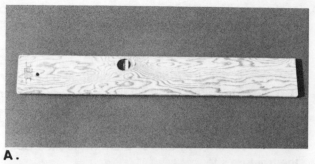

A.

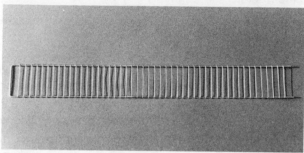

B.

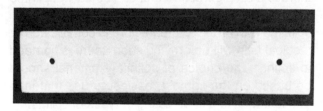

C.

D.

Figure 5-4. *Improvised splints.*

A. Longer boards are useful for fractured legs.

B. Wire-ladder splints can be bent into different shapes to contour with injuries. Covering the wire provides padding and greater comfort.

C. A padded wire-ladder splint.

D. Short boards can be used to splint arms, hands or fingers.

Soft splints. Pillows and blankets are often referred to as soft splints. They will mold around the limb and can be secured snugly with cloth ties. This type of splinting provides a soft, comfortable splint. Soft splints are also a good choice for large areas which need to be filled. For example, in splinting a fractured hip where the legs must be bound together, pillow or blankets are appropriate. Soft splints do not provide a great deal of support but are cheap and easily accessible.

Rigid splints. Boards and books are referred to as rigid splints. These are applied in the same manner as the soft splints, but provide more support while lacking the flexibility to to be molded around troublesome areas. Rigid splints are needed where fractured bone ends will move without firm support. When using boards or wood as improvised rigid splints, remember to pad the splint adequately before applying.

Commercially Prepared Splints

Pneumatic Splints. These are clear plastic inflatable devices which are also referred to as "air splints." Air splints are especially good to use with fractures where there is also light hemorrhaging. The bleeding wound may be dressed, and the air splint will provide a pressure dressing. An advantage of the air splint is that it allows for visual monitoring of the injury site; thus, if hemorrhaging continues, it can be detected and treated more quickly.

Wire ladder splints. These splints are made from lightweight metal frames which may be molded to limbs. This type of splint is useful for fractures which must be splinted without moving the injured limb, such as severely angulated fractures which require immobility.

Traction. These splints are used to stabilize femur fractures or severely angulated fractures of the lower leg. Traction splints may also be used to stabilize open fractures of the leg or lower leg and prevent the muscles of the thigh from drawing the bone ends together.

Commercial splints are simpler to apply and are more versatile than improvised splints, but both procedures should be mastered. Commercial splints are not always available when an emergency occurs, and not everyone can afford to buy them.

FIRST AID FOR SPECIFIC FRACTURES

Fractures of the Skull. Fractures of the skull are obviously dangerous because of the possibility of damage to the brain. In moving or transporting a victim with a suspected skull fracture, it is important to minimize the pressure placed on the fracture site. Position the victim on the side opposite the injury when possible. It is also important to properly dress and bandage all wounds associated with skull injury to keep them as clean as possible. Use sterile dressings and great care, since brain infections are very serious.

Fractures of the Face. Fractures of the face carry two possible complications beyond those expected with other fractures. First, if enough force was generated to fracture bones of the face, the same force may have caused injury to the cervical spine. Given this possibility, assume all victims of facial fractures suffer from cervical spine injury as well. A second possible complication with facial fractures is that sinuses may be hemorrhaging and blood entering the throat may be aspirated. In facial fractures, be especially careful to monitor the airway.

Fractures of the Spinal Column. Injuries which occur to the spinal column are extremely dangerous. Injuries to the spine may result in *paraplegia*, *quadraplegia* or even death. Injuries to the spine are usually to the cervical or lumbar vertebrae. These injuries are normally the result of *deacceleration injuries* (to the cervical spine) or *blunt trauma* (which occurs frequently to both areas). What makes spinal injuries even more important is that they may be made much worse by improper handling by the care giver. Caring for spinal injuries is difficult and requires special skills.

A thorough head-to-toe survey will alert the emergency caregiver to the possibility of spinal injuries. The most obvious sign occurs when the victim has no sensation in his or her extremities. Poor muscle control, loss of bowel or bladder control, or even tingling or dulled sensation in arms and legs are also signs of possible injury to the spinal column. If there are any signs of such injury or even suspicion of any signs, steps should be taken to prevent further injury.

If there are signs of injury evident in the chest and arms, an injury to the cervical (neck) spine should be suspected. If the chest and arms are okay, but the legs or lower abdomen show signs, an injury to the thoracic (chest area) or lumbar (lower back) spine should be suspected. *Regardless of the location of the suspected injury, the spine must be immobilized. Further injury is likely if the spine is allowed to move.*

For injuries that may include the neck, begin with application of gentle traction on the head in order to stabilize the neck. This will help steady the cervical spine. A stiff neck brace should be used (Fig. 5-5 shows three different types of cervical collars). Do not release traction until the victim's spine has been immobilized. For spinal injuries of any location, the use of a backboard or other firm support is absolutely necessary.

To place a victim on a backboard use the log roll maneuver. This process requires at least three rescuers; if they are not available, do not move the victim until they can be located. Untrained people can help, but you must train them using an uninjured simulated victim. *Remember, you only get one chance. Practice first, then place the victim on the backboard.* One rescuer must maintain control of the cervical spine by exerting gentle traction on the head. The other two or three rescuers should position themselves alongside the victim; one near the shoulders, one at the hips, one near the knees. The rescuer is in a position to see the actions of all the other rescuers and can maintain the spine at the same time. On her command, the victim is rolled onto his or her side and the backboard positioned underneath. Again, on command of the rescuer at the head, the victim should be carefully lowered onto the backboard. If not correctly positioned, it will be possible to slide the victim without moving the spine. Once correctly positioned, the victim can be secured onto the backboard with cravats. Blankets or sandbags can be used to secure the head and cervical spine.

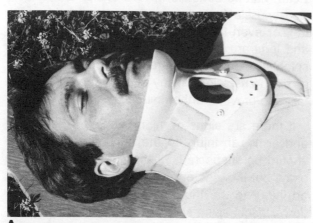

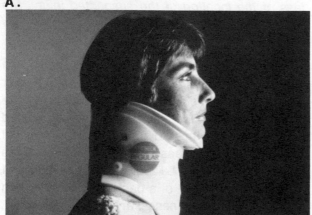

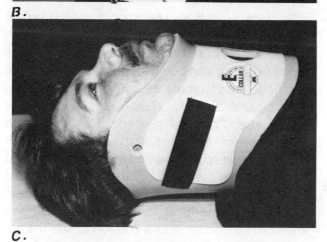

Figure 5-5. *Cervical collars.*

A. *A Philadelphia Cervical® collar.*

B. *The Stiffneck® collar.*

C. *The E-® collar.*

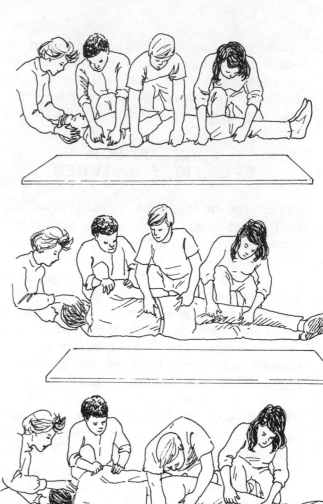

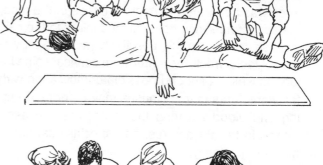

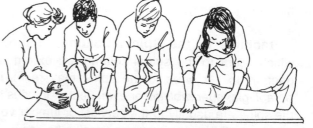

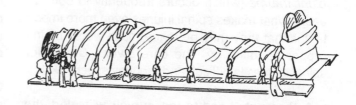

Figure 5-6. *Application of a full backboard.*

Fractures of the Clavicle. When the clavicle is fractured, the shoulder that is held in place will droop downward toward the front. Splinting helps support the arm and reduces pressure on the shoulder. Support may be most efficiently and easily supplied by application of a sling and swathe. (See Fig. 5-7 and 5-8.) Tie a simple knot at the apex of a triangular bandage to make a cup for the elbow. Lay the end of the triangular bandage closest to the body over the shoulder opposite the injury. Pull the other end of the triangular bandage over the other shoulder and tie off on the side of the neck.

Fractures of the Scapula. Scapula fractures are best treated with a sling and swathe. Diagnosis of this type of fracture is made by observation of point tenderness and painful movement of the shoulder. Scapula fractures are uncommon and are usually associated with a direct blow

Fractures of the Humerus. Fractures of the humerus result in tenderness at the fracture site, swelling and discoloration. Some fractures of the humerus result in nerve damage, and neurological or circulatory deficiency, which may be assessed by checking the radial pulse. Check distal pulse and if absent or diminished, apply light manual traction before splinting. To apply manual traction firmly grasp the arm well above and below. Now pull firmly from below the break using the site above the fracture as a point of resistance. (See Fig. 5-9.)

Fractures of the Elbow. With fractures of the elbow there may be a great deal of pain, swelling and possible deformity. It is imperative that the elbow not be moved more than absolutely necessary in splinting; therefore, wire ladder or soft splints are called for. These splints can be molded around the fracture without moving the area. It is always necessary to check circulation and neurological function with fractures, but especially so with fractured elbows.

Fractures of the Forearm. As with most fractures, the symptoms and signs of forearm fractures are point tenderness, swelling and deformity with discoloration. With severe fractures to the rad-

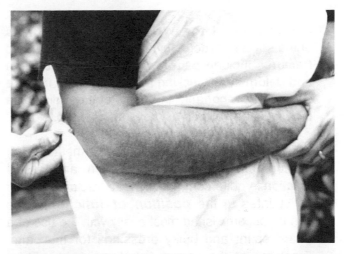

Figure 5-7. *Sling.*

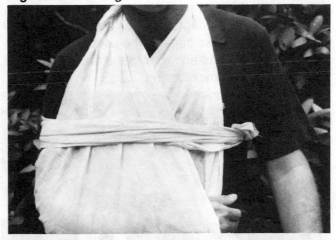

Figure 5-8. *Sling and swathe.*

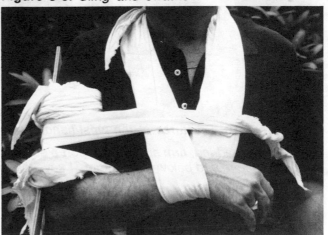

Figure 5-9. *Humerus splint.*

dius or ulna there may also be shortening of the limb. Air splints are useful for simple fractures of the forearm, but the sling and swathe are just as effective.

117

Fractures of the Wrist/Hand. Regardless of the specific bone(s) involved, most wrist or hand fractures include pain, swelling, loss of function and deformity. Checking pulse below the fracture site is very important. In breaks of the radius/ulna they must be splinted as they lie. (See Fig. 5-10.)

Fractures of the hand (carpals and metacarpals) produce extreme swelling and pain, and loss of function is quite common. These fractures should be splinted in the *position of function*. This can be accomplished most easily with the use of a board splint and bulky dressings for the palm. Fractures of the fingers (*phalanges*) should be splinted using a pliable aluminum splint if available. Padded tongue depressors or equivalently sized and shaped sticks can also be used. As a last resort, bind the broken finger to the one next to it for support and immobilization.

care in a comfortable position where breathing is easiest. If the victim cannot become comfortable, an arm may be strapped across the side of the chest on which the fracture occurred. The arm should be secured with wide strips of cloth or binding.

The exception to the non-threatening nature of rib fracture is the occurrence of three or more consecutive ribs which have been fractured in two or more places each. This condition is referred to as a **flail chest.** The flail chest is dangerous because as the chest wall rises during inspiration, the area of ribs which is fractured moves in the opposite direction. This is known as **paradoxical breathing.** Paradoxical breathing causes broken and detached areas of ribs to be pushed against pleura

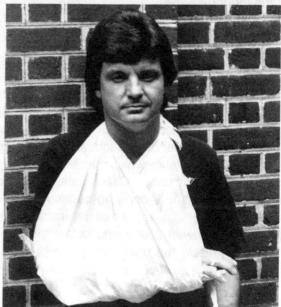

A.   **B.**

Figure 5-10. *Fractures of the wrist/hand.*

A. Use a padded, firm splint to support a suspected wrist/hand fracture. Attach the arm and hand to the board above and below the fracture. Leave the fingers in the position of function.

B. Complete the wrist/hand splint with a sling.

Fractures of the Ribs. Rib fractures are most commonly discovered by point tenderness and pain resulting from movement of the chest wall during breathing. The danger with rib fractures occurs when ribs are pushed into the muscles, pleura or lungs. For this reason the best treatment for broken ribs is to transport the victim to medical

and lungs. Another danger of paradoxical breathing is the inefficiency of respiratory efforts which become quite fatiguing.

Paradoxical breathing creates a great deal of pain during breathing, and may also lacerate other structures in the chest.

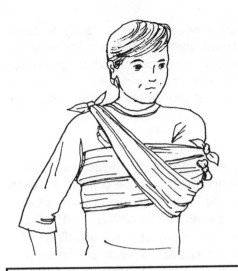

1. Place arm of injured side across chest.

2. Bind arm to chest with wide cravat.

3. Repeat with two additional cravats, overlapping bandages slightly.

4. Tie fourth cravat along angle of arm for support.

Figure 5-11. *First aid for rib fractures.*

Treatment of the flail chest injury requires the restriction of the injured side of the chest wall. Bulky material such as trauma dressings should be used to fill the void created during paradoxical breathing. If available, a sand bag is the ideal choice. The bulky material should be securely fixed over the injury site. Wide swathes are used to tie material in place. Swathes should be pulled tight while the victim exhales deeply. If the bandage is tied in place while the victim inhales, the result will be a loose bandage which will not restrict the movement of the chest wall.

Once immobilized, the flail chest victim should be transported on the injured side because of the danger of flail chest injury to chest cavity structures during paradoxical breathing. Because of this danger, chest movement must be minimized.

It is important to note that although rib fractures are more uncomfortable than dangerous in most cases, there are very real dangers associated with broken ribs. If broken ribs penetrate the muscles of the chest, one or more of the following may result.

Hemothorax. A hemothorax results in bleeding into the chest cavity causing pressure against the lung. The hemorrhage may be the result of trauma to the chest which results in laceration of blood vessels in the chest, or the result of penetrating injuries which lacerate vessels. The resultant hemorrhage causes blood to accumulate in the thoracic cavity, hindering the lungs' ability to expand. If unchecked, this may eventually cause the lung to collapse.

Pneumothorax. Pneumothorax occurs when air escapes into the thoracic cavity causing pressure to build up and the lungs to compress. The loss of air into the thoracic cavity outside the lungs may be the result of a chronic weak spot on the lung which finally bursts allowing gases from the lung to leak out. Another cause may be traumatic injury which lacerates the lung. Like hemothorax, if this condition persists, there will be a pressure build up in the thoracic cavity which may eventually result in collapse of the lung or progress into a more serious condition known as tension pneumothorax.

Sucking Chest Wound. Occasionally the mechanism of injury which fractured the ribs will also lacerate the chest wall. It is also remotely possible that the ribs could lacerate the chest wall. In any event, if there is a laceration of the chest wall, it is probable that a sucking chest wound would develop.

A sucking chest wound indicates that the chest wall has been lacerated; gases from the thoracic cavity are lost during exhalation; and atmospheric gases are pulled into the thoracic cavity during the inhalation phase. This condition is easily diagnosed as there will be a whistling sound during inhalation and **frothy** blood at the wound site.

Tension pneumothorax. Tension pneumothorax develops as a result of pressure within the chest cavity causing vital organs to be compressed and moved. This condition may result from spontaneous pneumothorax, collapse of part of the lung, or the result of a tightly dressed sucking chest wound.

In any case, there would be a buildup of pressure within the chest cavity. In the sucking chest wound one would only have to lift a corner of the bandage which occludes the wound to relieve the pressure. In the spontaneous pneumothorax, measures beyond this level of training are necessary to relieve the pressure.

In addition to collapsed lungs as in pneumothorax, there is a chance of bending the aorta as a result of moving the heart. Since the heart is suspended by ligaments in the chest cavity, it is vulnerable to movement because of the pressure build-ups we have discussed previously. The final result of tension pneumothorax then would be **cardiac insufficiency**—collapsed lung and death.

The important thing to remember about these emergencies is that they are life-threatening and there is little that can be done by an emergency care giver. Therefore, it is extremely important that the situation is recognized early, the victim is stabilized and quickly transported to a hospital.

Fractures of the Pelvis. Generally, a fracture of the pelvis is detected during the secondary survey. As the wings of the pelvis are compressed, the victim will react with pain if there is a fracture of the pelvis. If a fractured pelvis is suspected, immediate concern about hemorrhage is needed. The hemorrhage from a broken pelvis can result in sufficient blood loss to cause deep shock.

Depending on the area of the pelvis that has been fractured, there may be additional symptoms. If the fracture is near the joining of the sacral spine and iliac region of the pelvis there will probably be lower back pain. If the ishiopubic bones are fractured, there will be pubic tenderness, especially if the victim is sitting. Blood in the urine would indicate that the bladder may have been lacerated or contused by the fracture. Remember that a force of sufficient strength to fracture a pelvis may have caused internal bleeding and/or internal organ damage; therefore, monitor vital signs closely.

Victims with suspected pelvic fractures must be transported to a medical unit on a rigid surface such as a spine board or door. Bulky material should be placed under the victim's knees to reduce the pressure on the pelvis and abdominal regions. The victim's upper and lower body should be immobilized and attached to the rigid surface for transport.

Fractures of the Femur. Fractures of the femur are easily detected, as the signs of a broken femur are gross deformity, angulation, severe swelling and rotated thigh muscles. Often these fractures are open with resultant bleeding. Because the femur is such a thick, strong bone it takes a great deal of force to fracture it. This extremely thick bone is also surrounded by some of the strongest muscles in the body and has a rich blood supply.

In the fractured femur, there are often concurrent muscle spasms that are very strong and potentially dangerous. Contraction of the quadriceps muscles is of sufficient strength to force the bone ends of the fractured femur into the muscle and perhaps even out of the thigh. Given this set of circumstances, it is easy to understand why a fracture of the femur can be so dangerous.

In many open femur fractures, the bone will recede into the thigh; this fracture is still considered open. Blood loss in a fractured femur may total as much as one to two liters of blood so that moderate to severe shock is a possibility. If there is hemorrhage associated with a broken femur, it must be treated before splinting is undertaken. It is also important to remember the need for cleanliness.

When the femur is fractured, there is a great deal of pain for the victim. Pain is a contributing factor in shock. In the fractured femur, the combination of blood loss and pain creates a situation which makes shock a very real possibility.

Splinting for fractures of the femur is accomplished by the use of traction splints. There are several good commercial traction splints available and with a few supplies, a quite adequate improvised traction splint can be made. No matter which type of splint you use, there are a few general rules concerning traction splinting to keep in mind:

A. Apply *traction* only until the victim expresses relief from pain.

B. Apply traction only until both legs are about the same length.

C. If visible, traction must be discontinued when the bone starts to recede into the thigh.

D. Be especially careful not to release traction once it is applied as the tissue damage can be great.

The following is a step-by-step description of how to apply a commercially available traction splint (Figure 5-12):

1. One person applies manual traction being careful not to block access to the heel and top of the foot.

2. The splint is laid out and the length adjusted so that it goes from the victim's ischium to about one foot beyond the heel.

3. Adjust the elastic support straps so that they are above and below the knee, paying close attention that none of the straps goes over the knee.

4. Apply the ankle hitch. Apply traction by pulling on the straps and rings. Be sure to support the leg above and below the fracture site.

5. Place the splint under the victim so that the half ring is just below the buttock. Pad the groin and apply the strap to secure the ring.

6. Atach the ankle hitch to the splint and adjust the tension. Remember to apply the general rules of traction splinting.

7. Apply the velcro straps to stabilize the leg on the splint.

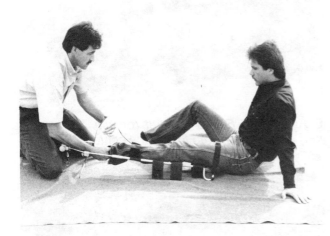

A.

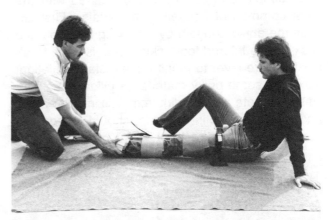

B.

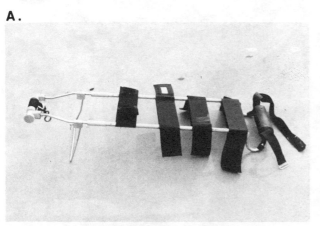

C.

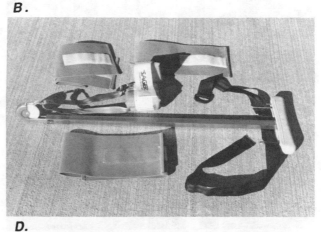

D.

Figure 5-12. **A**, applying a Hare® Traction splint and **B**, applying a Sager® Emergency Tracton splint. **C**, the Hare® Traction splint and **D**, the Sager® Emergency Tracton splint.

Fractures of the Lower Leg. The bones of the lower leg are the tibia and the fibula. Fractures of the lower leg usually result in both the tibia and fibula being broken. Either may be broken independently of the other, but if this is the case, usually the fibula is the single fracture. Due to its symmetry, most fractures of the tibia occur in the lower one fourth of the bone. (See Fig. 5-13.)

Signs of lower leg fracture are severe angulation, deformity, swelling and pain. These fractures are often open and the general rules of treatment for an open fracture apply. The treatment of choice for a complicated lower leg fracture of this type is traction splinting.

Fractures of the Ankle/Foot. Since fractures of bones in the foot and ankle are many times indistinguishable from sprains, it is best to treat all injuries as if they are fractures. Management is quite simple and can be accomplished with the most common of household materials. First expose the ankle and foot by removing the shoe and sock on the injured foot/ankle. This is done to allow the care giver to monitor the distal circulation. Next use some bulky material (a pillow does very well) to create a soft splint immobilizing the ankle and foot. The splint material should extend beyond the end of the heel about one foot. The splint should first be tied around the lower leg making sure the knots are over the remaining material extending beyond the heel should be pulled up against the sole of the foot and this should be tied around the foot. As in all fractures the injured foot/ankle should be elevated. (See Figs. 5-14 and 5-15.)

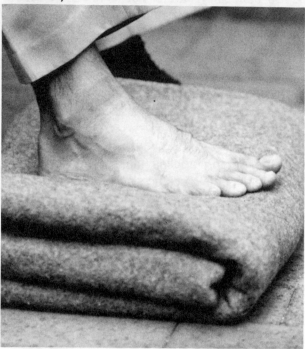

Figure 5-14. *Fold a blanket (or use a large pillow) and place injured foot in the center.*

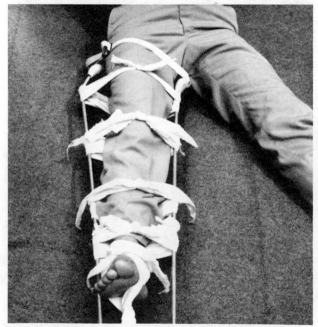

Figure 5-13. *Splint for a lower leg fracture.*

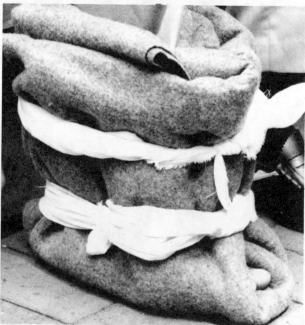

Figure 5-15. *Fold the blanket around the injured leg and secure with cravats. Elevate to control pain and swelling.*

STRAINS, SPRAINS AND DISLOCATIONS

Strains, sprains and *dislocations* are injuries to the joints. Joints are points of **articulation** between bones. Where bones come together there is a need for stability as well as motion. Ligaments hold bones in place at the articulation of joints. In the same way that bones must be held in place to function properly, muscles must have points of attachment at the origin (beginning) and insertion (termination) of the muscles to function properly.

If a joint is pressured to bend in an unnatural position, the ligaments which hold the bone ends in place may be stretched or torn. This is referred to as a sprain. If a muscle is stretched beyond its limits or taxed before it is stretched, the tendons which form the attachment may be torn. This condition is known as a strain. Occasionally, an articulation may be stressed to the point that the bone ends become displaced. This is referred to as a dislocation.

The symptoms for a sprain and a strain are very similar. A sprain is identified by the presence of swelling, discoloration, point tenderness and reduced mobility of the joint, and a strain is diagnosed by the presence of swelling, discoloration and pain.

Of course, one of the best ways to differentiate between strains and sprains is location. If the swelling and discoloration are in the joint, the injury is most likely a strain.

The only way to tell conclusively the difference between sprains, strains and fractures is by x-ray. Because of the difficulty in distinguishing among these three injuries, it is best to treat them all as though they were fractures. Emergency caregivers should always strive to err on the conservative side.

In a dislocation, bone ends are not in line at the joint. Ligaments must stretch and/or tear to allow the bone to be moved. Along with a great deal of pain, the result will be swelling and discoloration. These are the symptoms of any sprain or strain. In addition to the ligament and tendon damage, the rescuer may see gross deformity such as bone ends pressing against the skin.

Dislocations are dangerous for a number of reasons. First, a great deal of damage is done to the joint. Second, the displaced bone ends may compress and obstruct the flow of blood if the bone comes to rest against a blood vessel. Finally, the displaced bone end may put pressure on nerves at the dislocation site. It is important to protect against any unnecessary movement of a dislocation to reduce the risks of circulatory or neurologic damage.

Figure 5-16. *Splinting a dislocation.*

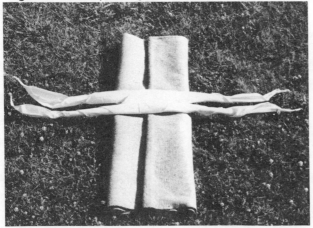

A. A quick and easy splint for a shoulder dislocation begins with a blanket and triangular bandages.

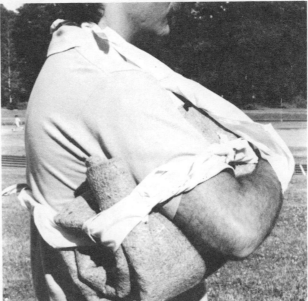

B. Use the blanket to maintain position and the triangular bandages to secure the arm. A third triangular bandage can be used as a wrist sling.

Building Skills: Splinting

Splints are important tools of the emergency caregiver. Properly used, they will prevent further injury and ease discomfort. To develop skills and gain proficiency in splinting, the rescuer should begin with a clear understanding of the skeletal anatomy of the body. To help develop these skills efficiently, begin by reviewing the anatomy section of the first chapter.

Directions: In groups of three to five, simulate appropriate first aid procedures for the injuries listed below. For each injury, apply the correct splint(s) and specify how circulation distal to the fracture can be assured. For each situation, have one group member assume primary responsibility for deciding how to treat the victim, with other members being asked to assist if necessary. At least one group member should act as an observer, and make notes to provide feedback to the caregivers.

PROFICIENCY

Satisfactory   Recheck

1. Closed fracture of the clavicle
Arm sling   _____   _____
Cravat (swathe)   _____   _____
Circulation checked by   _____   _____
Comments of observer _____

_____

_____

2. Closed fracture of the humerus
Arm sling   _____   _____
Cravat (swathe)   _____   _____
Circulation checked by   _____   _____
Comments of observer _____

_____

_____

3. Elbow fracture, held at 30 degree angle by victim
Circulation checked by   _____   _____
Rigid splint(s)   _____   _____
Wrist sling   _____   _____
Cravat (swathe) (optional)   _____   _____
Recheck circulation   _____   _____
Comments of observer _____

_____

_____

4. Open fracture of forearm/wrist

Bleeding controlled by _____ _____

Bandage used _____ _____

Rigid splint, position of function _____ _____

Arm sling _____ _____

Circulation checked by _____ _____

Comments of observer _____

_____

_____

5. Flail chest, coughing up blood

Cravats applied _____ _____

Tighten when victim exhales _____ _____

First aid to help Breathing _____ _____

Comments of observer _____

_____

_____

6. Open fracture of femur

Application of manual traction _____ _____

Bleeding control _____ _____

Bandage of open wound _____ _____

Application of traction splint _____ _____

Circulation checked by _____ _____

Treatment for shock _____ _____

Comments of observer _____

_____

_____

7. Dislocation of shoulder

Allows victim to hold in most comfortable position _____ _____

Application of soft splint _____ _____

Sling _____ _____

Cravat (swathe) _____ _____

Circulation checked by _____ _____

Comments of observer _____

_____

_____

8. Severe sprain of ankle

Application of soft splint   _____   _____

Elevation   _____   _____

Circulation checked by   _____   _____

Comments of observer _____

_____

_____

9. Dislocation of thumb

Application of rigid splint   _____   _____

Elevation   _____   _____

Circulation checked by   _____   _____

Comments of observer _____

_____

_____

10. Suspected cervical spine injury

Head-to-toe survey   _____   _____

Application of traction   _____   _____

Assembly of group of rescuers   _____   _____

Log roll of victim onto backboard   _____   _____

Correct securing of victim   _____   _____

Application of cervical collar if available   _____   _____

Comments of observer _____

_____

_____

Chapter Six

Emergency Transport: Preventing Further Injury

In situations where professional help is not available and there is danger of further injury, or when a victim must be transported to medical attention, the emergency caregiver is faced with the challenge of moving the victim without making injuries worse.

This chapter presents information about emergency rescue and transportation as three main topics: (1) basic principles and techniques for moving victims; (2) techniques for moving and transporting victims using litters and commonly available household items; and (3) emergency procedures to be used for moving the injured under press of time or circumstances.

BASIC PRINCIPLES

It has been emphasized throughout this book that emergency caregivers should not move victims unless necessary. When it becomes necessary to move an accident victim, forethought and planning make the task safer for the victim and easier for the rescuer. The following principles should serve as a guide in moving victims.

1. As always, the ABCs come first. Insure an open airway, breathing and circulation before moving the victim.

2. Try to move the victim along the long axis of the body and in a straight line. Avoid any movements that cause twisting or turning.

3. Plan ahead so that the victim only needs to be moved once.

4. Plan transport so that breathing and heartbeat can be continuously monitored. If using a stretcher, for example, transport the victim feet-first so the rear stretcher-bearer can see the victim's face at all times.

5. Rehearse all maneuvers for transport and make certain that all rescuers know their roles before moving the victim.

Using Improvised Materials

Commercially available splints, stretchers, and other devices for transportation were discussed in Chapter 5. In many instances, however, the rescuer must improvise equipment for transporting the injured.

Many household items can serve this purpose well. Blankets and garden implements—hoes, shovels and rakes—can be used to make a litter. A ladder can also serve as a litter. A garden hose can be used as a rope to drag the victim. An ironing board may be used as a full backboard for a child or a partial backboard for an adult. In an emergency, the rescuer needs to consider the resources available in the immediate surroundings and improvise!

Using Untrained Help

In many instances a victim will need to be moved and the emergency caregiver will not have trained people on hand. Volunteer help can be useful in such situations. Quick orientation to the task and rehearsal are the keys to successful use of untrained volunteer help.

Orient volunteers to the task by demonstrating what they are being asked to do and having them practice on an uninjured person. Be sure that each volunteer understands what he or she is being asked to do and that the volunteer is able to carry out the task successfully. Before you move the victim, take time to assure the victim that the volunteers have been shown how to help and that you are confident they are able to do their jobs well.

LIFTS AND CARRIES

Three-Person Lift and Carry

Three rescuers can provide a satisfactory lift and carry in many situations. If the victim is large, however, three people will probably be insufficient to manage safely.

The ideal situation for the three-person lift occurs when there is no spinal injury, the victim is small to average in size and weight, and the rescuers are average to large in size. When using the three-person lift, insure that the person with responsibility for the victim's head has sufficient strength to carry out the lift safely.

> **In all cases, be sure that each rescuer places the knee nearest the victim's head or feet on the ground before lifting. This will help produce an even lift.**

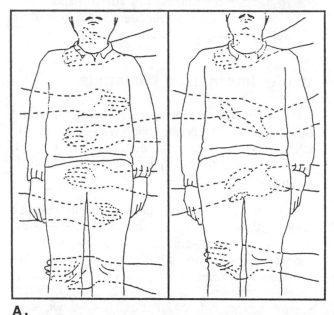

A.

Figure 6-1. *Three-person Lift and Carry.*

A. *Correct placement of hands beneath the victim.*

B. *The rescuer with the greatest strength is positioned near the parts of the body weighing most. Each rescuer should place the same knee on the ground in order to lift evenly.*

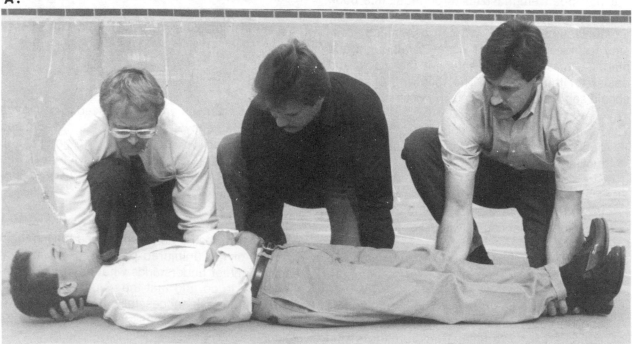

B.

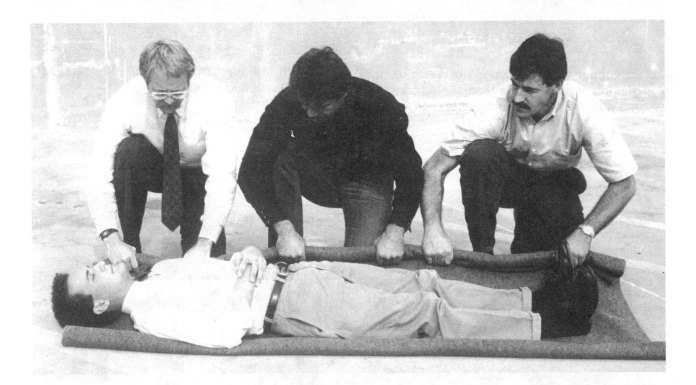

Figure 6-2. *The Blanket Lift. Three additional rescuers also lift from the near side of the blanket.*

Blanket Lift

Placing the victim on a solid object such as a backboard will make lifting relatively safe. When a backboard or other firm source is not available, a blanket may be used.

Using Litters

Litters can be carried by two or four rescuers. Two rescuers, one each front and back, is the method of choice. The remaining rescuers can walk on each side of the litter, monitor the victim and steady the litter if necessary. To make a smooth ride for the victim, the rescuers should

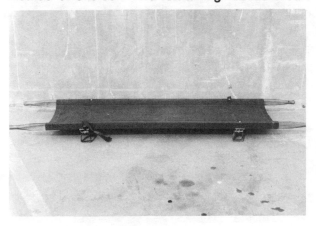

A.

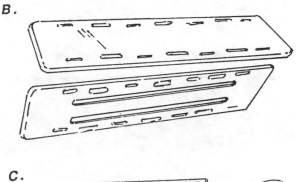

B.

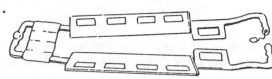

C.

Figure 6-3. *Types of litters: **A,** standard litter; **B,** long backboard; **C,** split frame (scoop) stretcher.*

walk with opposite feet leading. In starting off, for example, the rescuer in the lead should take the first step with the right foot while the rear rescuer starts with the left. This procedure will prevent side-to-side rocking of the litter.

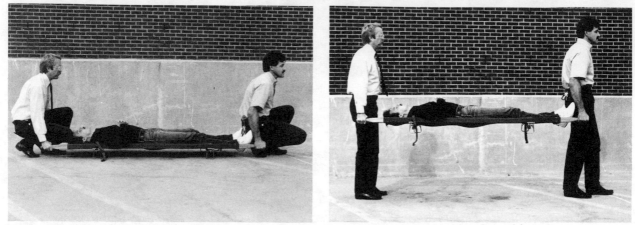

Figure 6-4. *Carrying the litter feet first allows the rescuer in the rear to monitor breathing.*

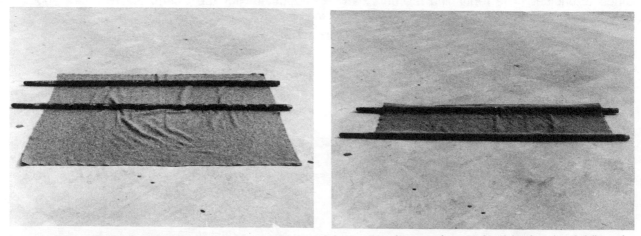

Figure 6-5. *An improvised litter can be constructed from two long poles and a blanket by folding the blanket around the poles. The weight of the victim will keep the litter together.*

WHEN THERE IS NO TIME

Rescuing injured victims trapped inside burning buildings, in automobiles on the verge of exploding, or in buildings about to collapse requires courage and skill. Courage is needed to attempt the rescue, but skill is essential to carry out the rescue without causing further injury to the victim. There is little time for thorough surveys—the rescuer must act quickly and responsibly with very little information.

Guidelines for reasonable actions in such emergency situations include:

1. Insure an open airway, provide rescue breathing, if needed, and maintain circulation of blood. If the victim has no heartbeat or is not breathing, then emergency rescue must be extremely quick if life is to be preserved. Once the victim has been moved to safety, CPR must begin immediately.

2. Maintain proper alignment of spine and limbs at all times.

3. Protect yourself from injury—an injured rescuer cannot help others effectively. Wait for help if at all possible.

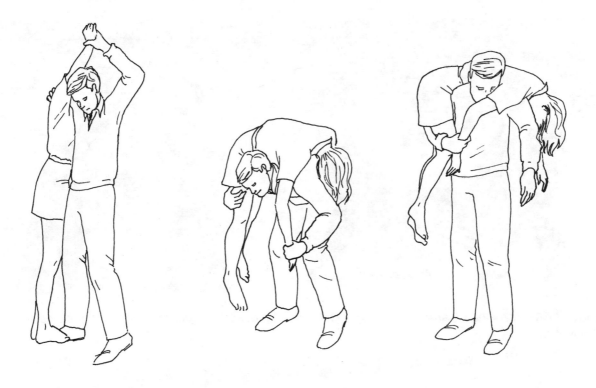

Figure 6-6. *The Fireman's Carry.*

RESCUE TECHNIQUES

When speed is critical, moving an injured or unconscious victim can be done in a number of ways. Transporting the victim on an improvised litter is a method of choice, followed by dragging, and, if necessary, carrying the victim in your arms.

Doors, pieces of plywood, or even chairs, may serve as improvised litters. For unconscious victims, use a firm, flat litter, such as a door. Carefully drag the victim onto the surface and then move. For conscious victims, a chair can be used for quick transportation.

> Lift with your legs, not your back. Begin with your legs bent and your buttocks down. Never lift with your legs held straight.

Dragging may be necessary when the victim is unconscious or no materials are available for an improvised litter. Always drag the victim with the spine and limbs in alignment. Never allow the spine to twist or bend. A blanket or rope can be very useful in dragging a victim, and can help to maintain alignment of spine and limbs.

When dragging is not feasible—flights of stairs are between the victim and safety, for example—and no other method of transport is available, the victim may have to be carried by the rescuer. Depending on the relative size of the victim and rescuer, the victim's injuries and state of consciousness, a fireman's carry or other hand carry may be used. (See Figure 6-6.)

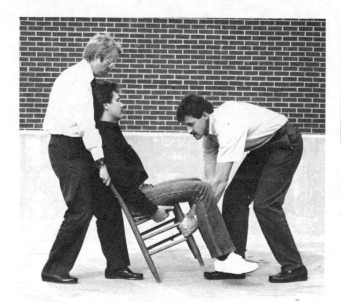
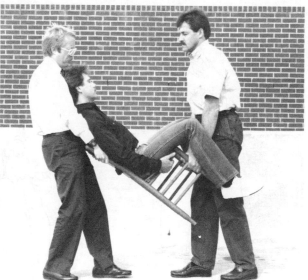

Figure 6-7. *The Chair Carry. This carry must never be used for a person with an injured pelvis, neck or back.*

BUILDING SKILLS

The skills necessary for safe rescue and transport of the injured are somewhat unique for emergency care. Rescue and transportation require communication with and management of groups of rescuers and occasionally on-the-spot teaching of untrained helpers. In some instances, the emergency caregiver must make decisions very quickly and remove the victim from a hazard without delay.

Directions: In groups of three to eight, simulate appropriate emergency rescue and/or transportation procedures for the situations listed below. For each situation, decide what must be avoided to prevent the victim from sustaining further injuries and provide transportation. For each situation, have one group member assume primary responsibility for deciding how to treat the victim, with other group members being asked to assist if necessary. At least one group member should act as an observer and make notes to provide feedback to the caregivers.

1. Your victim is breathing but unconscious. She has an obvious fracture of her left lower leg, but no other visible injuries. She is lying on the floor of a building that is on fire. The route to safety does not involve stairs.

PROFICIENCY

Satisfactory   *Recheck*

Log roll onto blanket   _____   _____

Blanket drag to safety   _____   _____

Assessment after reaching safety   _____   _____

Comments of observer   _____

_____

_____

2. Two individuals have been injured playing soccer. Both have painful ankle injuries. One chair is available, but due to time pressure, both must be taken to the infirmary at the same time.

Chair carry for one victim   _____   _____

For-and-aft carry for second victim   _____   _____

Comments of observer (s) _____

_____
Fore-and-aft

3. Your victim has been in a car wreck and has been thrown free. She is curled up in fetal position and claims to have no feeling in her legs. Gasoline is leaking from the car and it appears that it may explode any moment.

PROFICIENCY

Satisfactory   *Recheck*

Maintains spine alignment _____ _____

Places victim on board or blanket _____ _____

Instructs helpers as needed _____ _____

Transports safely _____ _____

Comments of observer (s) _____

_____

_____

4. Your victim has a serious injury and must be transported to a hospital. You have three untrained volunteers to work with in placing the victim on a litter.

Instruction to volunteers _____ _____

   lifting to be used _____ _____

   carrying on a litter _____ _____

   lifting to prevent jarring _____ _____

practice with uninjured volunteer _____ _____

four-person lift onto litter _____ _____

carry litter away _____ _____

Comments of observer (s) _____

_____

_____

Chapter Seven

Burns, Frostbite and Other
Temperature-Related Injuries

Our bodies are designed to operate within a relatively narrow range of temperatures. If internal temperatures vary too much, irreparable damage or even death may occur. To regulate temperatures, our bodies are designed with systems that allow for adjustments based on our activities and the environmental conditions outside.

In making temperature adjustments, the body treats itself as if it were composed of two separate parts, a core and a shell. The core includes the major internal organs (heart, brain, etc.), and the tissue immediately surrounding these structures. The shell includes things other than the vital functions: the skeleton, arms and legs, and the skin.

The body has an involuntary mechanism that works to keep the core temperature plus or minor one degree Fahrenheit. To regulate temperature the body can alter the amount of blood that is sent to the core or to the shell. When environmental temperature goes up, more blood is sent to the shell to carry excess heat to the skin where it can be released. The release can be accomplished through sweating and/or convection (release of heat into air). When temperatures are too low, on the other hand, blood is diverted away from the shell and into the core to preserve heat. This adjustment produces the characteristic blue skin that is associated with being cold. Another adjustment to cold is increased muscle activity such as "goose flesh" ("chill bumps") and shivering. Increased muscle activity also generates heat.

If environmental conditions are sufficiently extreme, body tissues may be damaged or destroyed by burning or freezing. Although the shell is the part of the body that is most visibly affected by extreme heat or cold, the core of the body is also affected. In this chapter, we will discuss how the emergency caregiver can use the concept of core and shell to guide first aid for burning and freezing emergencies. The emergency caregiver must attend to the damage done to the shell as well as to the body's need to preserve the core. The damage to the shell comes in the form of burns and frostbite. Body reactions which preserve the core and maintain its vital functions are often the result of burn shock, heat exhaustion, heat stroke and hypothermia.

BURNS

First aid is very important for burns and other heat-related injuries because, as is true with many other types of injuries, action that is taken soon after the accident can lessen the severity of the burn, speed recovery and help to limit disability. In many cases, lives may be saved by first aid measures.

Burn injuries are classified in several ways. Classification is an important part of assessment because first aid measures differ according to the type of burn.

The first classification of burns is based on the source of the burn: thermal, chemical, electrical

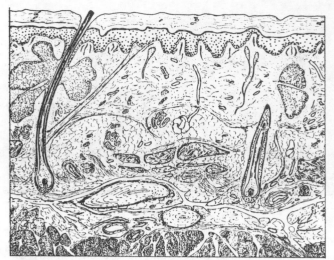

Figure 7-1. *Cross section showing layers of skin.*

and radiation. The second and third classifications for burns relate to the amount of surface area burned (extent), and the depth of tissue destruction (expressed as the *degree* of the burn — first, second and third).

Thermal burns occur when the body — or a part of the body — is exposed to extreme temperatures. Beyond 113 degrees (45 degrees Celsius) the cells of the body will die.

Chemical burns occur when the body participates in a chemical reaction with caustic substances. These caustic substances — strong acids or alkalines — have the ability to interact with the human body and dissolve it! The action of dissolving the body results in the burn.

Electrical burns occur when the body comes into contact with strong electrical current. As electricity passes from the source — a bare wire, a power line or a faulty appliance, for example — into the victim's body, resistance develops that results in burning of flesh. Electrical burns are only one problem with encountering a strong electrical current, though. The upset of the body's own electrical system due to the added current from the shock may cause the heart to stop beating and disrupt other ongoing body processes.

Radiation can also burn human flesh. Like electricity, radiation is a form of energy that can penetrate the human body. Resistance develops where this energy meets the skin and burning occurs. Sunburn develops, for example, when ultraviolet radiation burns the skin.

How Burns Cause Damage

Before discussing the types of burns and the first aid needed for each, it is important to understand how various body structures react to burning. As Figure 7-1 shows, the skin protects the body with a series of layers of cells. The skin is enormously important because it prevents harmful organisms from entering the body, seals in fluids that are vital to body functioning and has the capacity to sweat or shiver to help regulate the temperature inside the body. In most cases, the skin suffers the most serious damage from burns.

Depending on the depth of a burn, the damage to skin ranges from relatively minor, as in the case of sunburn where the outer layers of cells become burned, to life-threatening when all layers of skin are destroyed, the body loses fluid, and harmful microorganisms are not blocked from entering the body. Regardless of the cause or the depth of the burn, body tissues are destroyed. When the destruction occurs to a part that has the capacity to regenerate, such as the outer layers of the skin, the burn will usually heal completely. When the destroyed tissues cannot regenerate, as when all layers of skin are destroyed, scarring will occur.

Other body systems are also affected by burning. The respiratory system is very sensitive to extreme temperatures, caustic chemicals and radiation, for example. When the respiratory system is burned, swelling often occurs, making breathing difficult or impossible.

Given the fact that body systems are affected by burns directly or indirectly, the impact of burns on health are as follows:

Infection: If the skin is badly damaged by a burn, harmful microorganisms will have an easier time gaining a foothold in the body. The more skin damage there is, the greater the danger of infection. Additionally, given the fact that the body is injured, the ability to fight off the infection may be compromised because the body is also working to repair the burned tissues.

Shock: Serious burns commonly upset the fluid balance of the body. The body will rush plasma to the burn site, which often makes serious burns appear to be glistening with moisture. Losing sufficient plasma in this way can result in a serious fluid imbalance known as "burn shock."

Pain: Burns can be intensely painful, particularly when the nervous system is damaged but not destroyed. Curiously, the most serious types of burns (third degree) may be relatively painless, while those of lesser seriousness (first and especially second degree) may be very painful. Pain may cause or aggravate shock, in addition to having a dramatic emotional impact on the burn victim.

Thermal Burns

Thermal burns, burns caused by heat, are the most common type of burn injury. Heat can be transmitted to humans through a variety of means: fire, hot liquids, molten synthetic fabrics in clothing, steam, etc. Thermal burns are classified by *degree* and *extent*. Degree relates to the depth of tissue destruction: first, second and third degree. Extent refers to the amount of surface area of the body that is involved. The amount of surface area that is burned is important because survival from burns is directly related to the amount of surface area involved. The more surface area burned, the poorer the chance for survival. The degree of the burn also enters this equation. Second and third degree burns are much more threatening to survival than first degree burns. Other considerations aside, an individual with extensive first degree burns would have a better chance of survival than another person who might have less extensive burns of second and third degree.

First Degree Burns

First degree burns are those that involve the outer layer of skin only. Such burns are common, and will usually heal without complications. First degree burns have a characteristic appearance. The skin is reddened and may be mottled; it will very warm to the touch, and the victim will feel discomfort (pain) particularly where clothing rubs against the burned skin. Mild swelling may also develop.

Second Degree Burns

Burns that are classified as second degree involve destruction of deeper tissues than first degree. The hallmarks of second degree burns are blisters that develop at the burn site. The burn may also appear wet due to leakage of plasma. Swelling commonly occurs as well. Second degree burns can be intensely painful because nerve endings may have been severely irritated. Second degree burns are often more painful than more serious third degree burns because deeper burning may destroy nerve ends.

Third Degree Burns

Third degree burns involve destruction of skin and underlying tissues. Skin may be blackened with soot, but the burned tissue appears charred and coagulated (leathery). Third degree burns are very dangerous because of shock and the possibility of infection.

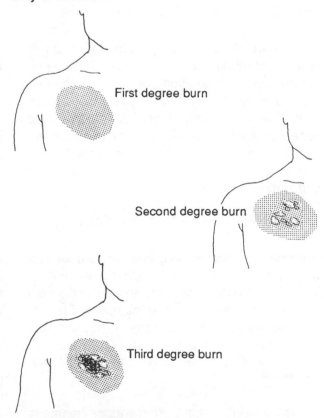

First degree burn

Second degree burn

Third degree burn

Figure 7-2. *Classifications of burns by degree.*

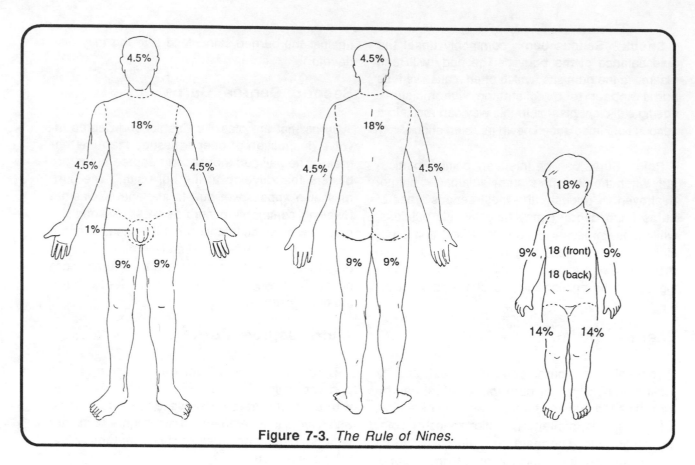

Figure 7-3. *The Rule of Nines.*

Estimating Size of Burned Area

The size or amount of body surface burned can be estimated using the *rule of nines*. This rule divides the body into sections of surface area that are all multiples of nine. (See Figure 7-3.) We can also use the rule of palms where the area covered by one palm =1%, so the number of palms required to cover a burn would represent the % burn area. This requires experience and is thus less useful to most first aiders.

First Aid for First Degree Burns

The primary objectives in giving first aid for first degree burns are to stop the burning and relieve pain. Stop the burning by removing the victim from the source of heat. Pain may be relieved by applying cool water. Submerge the burned surfaces in cool water until the pain subsides. Where submersion is not possible, gently apply cool, wet compresses.

There is no need to apply ointments or creams to burns. These substances act to hold in heat and may actually make the burn worse. Cool water is the best remedy.

First Aid for Second Degree Burns

As in the case of first degree burns, the immediate first aid objectives are to remove the individual from the source of the burn and relieve pain. An additional objective for second degree burns is to *avoid breaking blisters*.

Immerse the burned area in cool water until the pain subsides, taking care to avoid breaking any blisters that may have developed. For areas that cannot be immersed, cool, wet compresses may be used. In cooling the burned area(s), it is important to realize that it is likely that first degree burns will be present around the edges of the second degree burn. Treat first and second degree burns with cool water. When the cooling has eased the pain, a clean, dry dressing may be used to protect the second degree burn. The dressing should always be used if any of the blisters have broken. A dressing offers protection to unbroken blisters as well as a barrier to microorganisms. In choosing a dressing, be sure to select material that will not come apart if wet, such as absorbent cotton. Such material will adhere to the burned area, and removal will be exceedingly painful. When changing the dressing, which should be done if it begins to develop an odor or becomes soaked with body fluids, soak it off with large amounts of water. Never forcefully pull a dressing off a burn! The underlying tissue may come off with the dressing!

First Aid for Third Degree Burns

Third degree burns may present a life-threatening emergency. While first and second degree burns usually heal without extensive medical attention, with third degree burns the destruction of tissue is such that medical attention should always be sought. Attention to immediate medical needs, skin grafting for areas where skin has been burned off, and infection prevention and control must be aggressively pursued. Because of the seriousness of third degree burns, the objectives for first aid begin at the beginning. After removing the victim from the he source of the burn, make certain that the victim has an open airway and heartbeat. Begin treatment for shock at once. Objectives for treatment of the burned area include making certain that contamination of the burn is prevented, applying non-absorbent dressings and transporting the victim to a source of medical care that is equipped to deal with burn injuries (preferably a burn unit). If possible, immobilize and elevate the burned area to reduce swelling. Once again, do not break any blisters that may be present. It is common for serious burns to include first and second along with third degree.

Electrical Burns

Electric shocks have many effects, including stoppage of heartbeat in some cases and burns at the site where the body and the source of electricity made contact. First aid for electric burns includes the following objectives: safely break contact between the accident victim and the electricity, insure breathing and heartbeat, and attend to burns and other injuries.

Breaking contact between the accident victim and the source of electricity must be carried out with forethought because there is great danger of the rescuer getting shocked in trying to help. If the electricity cannot be shut off by unplugging an appliance or tripping a breaker, use a tool made of wood or other **non-conducting** (non-metal) material to break contact between the victim and the source of electricity. Do not touch the victim (or anything made of metal that the victim is touching) until contact with the source of the electric shock has been broken. Once contact has been broken, immediately assess the victim for breathing and pulse and begin artificial respiration or CPR as needed.

First aid for electrical burns is the same as for any other thermal burn. However, it is common to underestimate the extent of damage—all electrical burns are serious. There may be first, second and/or third degree burns present. Action to relieve pain, prevent and treat shock, and prevent infection should be taken without delay. Any victims of serious electric shock should be seen by a physician.

Chemical Burns

Chemical burns occur when the body takes part in a chemical reaction with a caustic acid or alkaline.

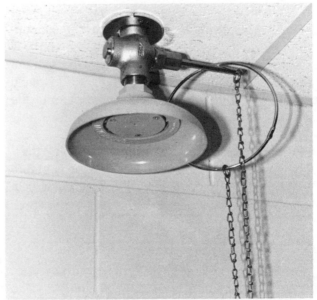

Figure 7-4. *Emergency showers such as the one shown here are useful for giving burn first aid.*

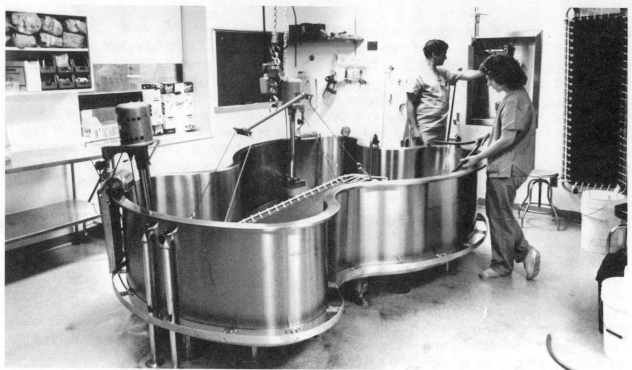

Figure 7-5. *Burn units in hospitals are capable of providing excellent care for victims of burns. Large tanks such as the one shown make it possible to treat the victim with a minimum of discomfort.*

Such burns can occur on the surface of the body, or internally through ingestion or inhalation. Objectives for first aid for chemical burns include first stopping the chemical reaction, followed by attention to the damage.

Water should be used to stop the chemical reaction. Using a shower or hose, wash the affected area(s) with water for at least 15 minutes. Stop the water and see if the burning resumes. If so, continue to wash with water until the burning has stopped. Remove any pieces of clothing with the caustic chemical on them, taking care to avoid spreading the chemical to unburned parts of the body.

If the burn is from **dry lime,** however, thoroughly brush the loose lime from the body before applying water. Water reacts with dry lime and heat is produced!

Radiation Burns

Burns from radiation may result from exposure to the sun (solar energy) or nuclear energy. Too much sun exposure results in sunburn. Such burns are usually first or second degree burns, and should be treated accordingly. Exposure to nuclear energy (ionizing radiation) is a different matter. Ionizing radiation cannot be seen or felt in the same way as heat from the sun may be felt. Ionizing radiation affects the cells of the body in many way, in addition to producing burns on the skin. Cells that normally divide often, such as those that line the stomach and intestines and those that produce hair, are most easily affected by ionizing radiation. Effects on other cells are difficult to predict, but may include genetic changes and cancer. The amount of damage from ionizing radiation depends on a number of factors, including the characteristics of the source of the radiation, and the duration and intensity of exposure.

The objectives for first aid for exposure to ionizing radiation are removing the victim from further exposure, removal and proper disposal of the victim's clothing that has been been contaminated, and transport of the victim to medical attention. The victim's clothing should be handled as little as possible, and the first-aider should seek assistance from public health authorities to determine the best means for safe disposal of contaminated material.

OTHER HEAT-RELATED INJURIES

Burns are not the only reaction of the body to exposure to excessive heat. The mechamisms within the body that regulate temperature are critical to health, and when they are exposed to stress they may break down. The three types of "breakdown" discussed here are heat exhaustion, heat cramps, and heat stroke.

Heat Exhaustion

Prolonged exposure to hot temperatures, particularly in high humidity, may lead to loss of water and salt that is so excessive that some individuals suffer what is known as heat exhaustion. The symptoms of this condition include the following:

1. weakness, dizziness, nausea
2. pale, cool and clammy skin
3. rapid and weak pulse
4. profuse sweating

Although heat exhaustion is rarely life-threatening, first aid is needed.

First Aid for Heat Exhaustion

Remove the victim from the hot environment if possible. Encourage the victim to lie down. Remove excessive clothing and protect the individual from exertion. Sponge with cool water. If the victim feels faint, elevate the feet and legs 8 to 12 inches. Give the victim sips of cool water. Give the water in sips at the rate of about half a glass (4 oz.) per 15 minutes. *Do not force liquids. Do not give liquids to victims who are nauseated or vomiting.* If the victim begins to feel nauseous, stop giving water immediately. The victim should be encouraged to avoid exercise for several days following the episode of heat exhaustion. Medical advice should be sought if there is any doubt about the victim's condition.

Heat Cramps

Heat cramps are usually associated with physical exertion in hot weather. Large muscle groups such as the legs are most commonly affected. When heat cramps strike, the affected muscle(s) go into spasm, causing severe discomfort. Mysteriously, cramps seem to occur more commonly in some individuals than others, and seem to be related to the balance of fluid and salt in the body. Although cramps may be prolonged and painful, they are normally not life threatening.

First Aid for Heat Cramps

Give 2-3 glasses of cool water sipped slowly. Manual massage of the cramping muscle(s) may

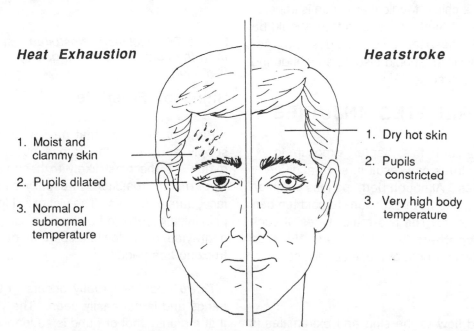

Figure 7-6. *Symptoms of heatstroke and heat exhaustion.*

Heat Exhaustion

1. Moist and clammy skin
2. Pupils dilated
3. Normal or subnormal temperature

Heatstroke

1. Dry hot skin
2. Pupils constricted
3. Very high body temperature

bring relief, although some experience greater discomfort from massage. Massage should be down and up the long axis of the bone.

Heat Stroke

Heat stroke differs from heat exhaustion and heat cramps in one very important way. Heat stroke is a potentially fatal condition. Heat stroke occurs when the temperature regulating mechanism of the body fails and body temperature increases. Without prompt treatment, the victim will suffer irreversible brain damage. Nearly all untreated victims of heat stroke die, and nearly half of those who are treated will die. The symptoms of heat stroke are as follows:

1. hot, dry skin that appears flushed (red)
2. rapid, strong pulse
3. rapid, deep breathing

First Aid for Heat Stroke

The most important objective for first aid for heat stroke is reducing body temperature as soon as possible. To reduce body temperature effectively, remove the victim's clothing and place him/her in a tub of cool water. If this is not possible, sponge with cool water. Continue until the temperature remains under 104 degrees F for an adult, 105 degrees F for a child. Medical attention is imperative for victims of heat stroke, and they should be transported to a hospital as soon as possible. Advice from a physician should also be sought during administration of first aid.

COLD-RELATED INJURIES

As stated earlier in this chapter, exposure to extreme temperatures can result in several different types of injuries. Although perhaps less common than burns, injuries from exposure to cold temperatures are serious. The two major types of such injuries are **hypothermia** and **frostbite**. First aid is very important for both of these conditions.

Frostbite

When blood flow to the skin and extremities is insufficient to maintain temperature, ice particles may form. This only occurs when the temperature of the environment outside the body is below freezing, of course. Frozen tissue is damaged, and the damage can be devastating in severe cases. Fortunately, though, frostbite usually develops relatively slowly, which means that first aid can be very effective in halting progression and reversing frostbite. The key to effective first aid for frostbite is early recognition of the signs of the condition — the same key as for hypothermia, as we shall see later.

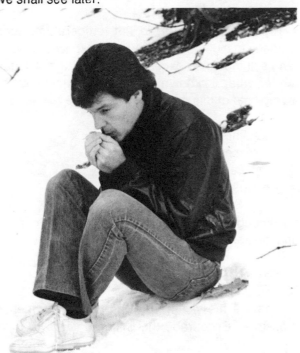

Figure 7-7. *Victims of frostbite must be removed from the cold environment quickly to prevent further injury.*

Signs of Frostbite

Parts of the body that have inadequate blood supply and those that are exposed to the elements are the most likely to become frostbitten. *Superficial* frostbite can usually be seen on the face, ears or fingers. The victim will feel tingling or pain initially, followed by numbness. The skin has a grayish or yellowish color in patches where freezing has begun.

Deep frostbite usually occurs in the feet and hands and is not easily seen. The victim reports that a painful foot or hand is suddenly numb. The skin is cold and waxy.

First Aid for Frostbite

In all cases of frostbite, the first-aider needs to protect the victim from further injury by getting him/her out of the cold environment. If this is not possible, and there is great risk that a thawed body part may become re-frozen, it is better to leave the body part frozen until it is possible to get the victim to safety. Protect a frostbitten body part by preventing the victim from using it in any way. Do not allow a person to walk on a frozen foot or toes, or use a frozen hand or finger. Any movement of frozen tissue will cause damage that will only become apparent when thawing takes place. Because frozen tissue is numb, the victim may become burned during rewarming. Protect victims from too much heat. Remember, alcohol does not help to maintain warmth. In fact, alcohol speeds cooling, because it generates a great deal of heat that must be shed by the body — by shunting blood to the skin. Thus the skin may feel warm, but the core temperature is being lowered. When all of the alcohol has been metabolized, the body temperature will be lowered.

For superficial frostbite on the face, ear or finger, a warm hand will effectively stop the freezing. Place a warm hand directly (gently) over the affected area. Remove the victim to safety as well. Give the victim warm drinks.

Deep frostbite requires more extensive first aid. Rapid rewarming in water (102 — 108 degrees F.) is recommended. Continue until the affected tissues are flushed red or bluish. This process should continue for 20 — 30 minutes at minimum. The victim will usually experience severe pain during thawing of deep frostbite. Give the victim hot drinks (non-alcoholic!). Once thawing is complete, encourage the victim to *gently* exercise the affected part. Do not break blisters if they develop, and separate fingers or toes with gauze pads. Reccomend that the victim of frostbite see a physician in all but superficial cases that are quickly thawed.

Hypothermia

Hypothermia means low core body temperature. This condition occurs when the body loses more heat than it is able to generate. Formerly referred to as "exposure", hypothermia may or may not be accompanied by frostbite.

Hypothermia is a very dangerous condition with a high mortality rate. As body temperature falls, mental processes are altered. As a result, the victim of hypothermia may not be aware of what is happening to him/herself. When body temperature falls below 90 degrees F., shivering ceases and the victim will slip into a coma and die.

First Aid for Hypothermia

The primary objective for first aid for hypothermia is to prevent further loss of heat from the victim. Get the victim out of wet clothes or, if not possible, cover with plastic (insulating underneath as well as on top) to preserve body heat. Give hot drinks if conscious and not nauseated, immerse in warm water (102 — 108 degrees F.) and use any other means to safely warm the victim. If the hypothermia is severe, CPR may be needed.

Curiously, hypothermia sometimes acts as a protective mechanism for exposure to severe cold. Sudden cooling of the body will sometimes make the victim lose heartbeat and respiration and appear dead. Such victims may be revived, though, and should be maintained with CPR.

Building Skills:
Decisions about Burns, Heat Injuries, Frostbite and Hypothermia

The skills developed from study of this chapter, as well as for those that follow, are different from previous chapters. Instead of requiring new performance skills, first aid for burns, heat injuries, frostbite and hypothermia is based on correct assessment of the condition of the victim and careful decisions about actions.

Directions: For each of the situations listed below, review the part(s) of the text that apply and develop a plan for delivering first aid.

a. Your victim's clothing is on fire. The first action is taken by a bystander who puts out the flames by rolling the victim on the ground. The victim's clothes are still smoldering as you approach. Of the pairs of procedures given, which should you do first? Why?

1. ABC survey or stop clothes from smoldering

_____

_____

2. Send for help or begin head-to-toe survey

_____

_____

3. Apply cold water compress or treat for shock

_____

_____

4. Estimate extent and depth of burns or treat for shock

_____

_____

b. Your victim has received a severe scalding burn to his face and neck from a broken steam pipe. Of the pairs of procedures given, which should you do first? Why?

1. ABC survey or apply cold water to burns

_____

_____

2. Send for help or apply cold water to burns

_____

_____

3. Position for better breathing or send for help

_____

_____

4. Position for better breathing or continue with cool water

_____

_____

c. Your victim is an elderly man who has collapsed on a street corner. He has a very red face, his skin is hot to the touch, and he appears to be slightly twitching. Of the pairs of procedures given, which should you do first? Why?

1. ABC survey or send for help

_____

_____

2. Head-to-toe survey or send for help

_____

_____

3. Begin treatment for shock or apply cool water

_____

_____

4. Monitor respiration and heartbeat or maintain body temperature

_____

_____

d. You are hiking in the woods in December. The wind is blowing and it is very cold. One of your party has greyish-white patches on his cheeks. When you ask how he feels he replies that he is just fine. Of the pairs of procedures given, which should you do first? Why?

1. Examine patches on face or wait awhile longer and reassess later

_____

_____

2. Ask victim other questions to determine mental status or cover patches with a hand or clothing.

_____

_____

3. Begin walking toward shelter or give victim shot of hard liquor to drink

_____

_____

4. Reassess patches on face or begin planning how to get victim to medical attention

_____

_____

e. Visiting an elderly friend in his home, you notice that the house seems cold. Your friend is somewhat disoriented today, generally sickly. The longer you visit, the more you notice these changes. Your friend does not complain of being cold, but is clearly not himself. Of the pairs of procedures given, which should you do first? Why?

1. Carry out a thorough head-to-toe survey or feel your victim's skin

_____

_____

2. Take your friend's temperature or give him a shot of liquor

_____

_____

3. Give your friend something hot to drink or urge him to get up and get moving.

_____

_____

4. Call for medical advice or try to stop being such a worrier

_____

_____

Chapter Eight

Poisonings

Poisonings are generally time-critical events. The longer a poison remains in the victim's stomach or bloodstream, the lower that victim's chances for survival. Because poisoning is a life-threatening event, it is important that you pay careful attention to the management of poisoning emergencies.

The term *poisoning* refers to the introduction of a harmful foreign substance into the body. The foreign substance may produce a wide variety of bodily reactions depending on what type of chemical is introduced. The victim may stop breathing, the heart may stop beating or beat irregularly, the kidneys or liver may stop functioning, or other body systems may fail. The term *overdose,* while meaning the same thing, implies intentional ingestion of a substance with the intent of harm.

Poison control centers have been established in or near large population centers. These centers compile lists of potentially poisonous substances and new products. These centers can then identify substances and how they must be treated. Generally this information is available to hospitals and physicians, but it is important for private citizens also. If medical help is a great distance away and something must be done immediately, then the poison control hotline is invaluable. It is a good idea for all homes to have the number of the poison control center near the phone.

In 1986, there were 5000 fatal, accidental poisonings, making poisoning the fifth most common cause of death. A large number of those accidental poisonings were to children who ingested poisonous substances in their home. The most common poisoning victim is under age eight. When a poisoning accident happens to a young victim, the situation is dangerous for more than one reason. First, the very young have limited communication abilities and may be able to offer no more than limited assistance in identifying the substance in question. Secondly, the very young suffer greater mortality from any situation which taxes the body's ability to overcome and repel assaults on bodily defenses.

Poisonous substances may be introduced into the body in a number of ways. Poisons may be breathed into the lungs *(inhaled)*, swallowed into the stomach *(ingested)*, passed through the skin *(contact)*, or be forced through the skin *(injected)*.

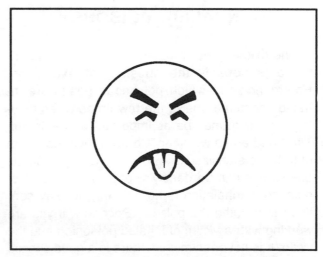

Figure 8-1. *The "Mr. Yuk" sticker was created as a friendly reminder to children not to touch any container bearing the sticker. The stickers may be obtained from area poison control centers.*

Poisons may also be thought of in terms of the types of changes they produce in the body. Changes in structure and function may be grouped as follows:

1. **Corrosives** — substances which destroy tissue directly, such as lye and ammonia.

2. **Irritants** — substances which cause inflammation of mucous membranes, such as arsenic.

3. **Nerve toxins** — substances which affect basic cell processes, including the narcotics and cocaine.

4. **Blood toxins** — substances which deprive the blood of oxygen; examples include carbon monoxide and carbon dioxide.

The management of poisonings is, at the same time, one of the easiest and one of the most difficult emergencies to deal with. It is easy because the rescuer most often must do three things: support respirations, insure adequate circulation, and remove the drug. It is difficult because of the uncertainty of knowing what and how the substance was ingested and knowing its unique characteristics.

INHALED POISONS

One of the major problems associated with inhaled poisons is the question of extrication. Emergencies in which poisonous gases are inhaled constitute one of the few times when moving the victim may be as important as treatment. Time and again we hear "Do not move the victim until he is stabilized." In dealing with poisonous gases, this can be deadly wrong! If the victim of poisonous inhalation is not moved, he may continue to breathe the poison. Secondly, if you are working with a victim of inhaled poisoning and the victim has not been moved, there is a good chance you are breathing the same poison and can eventually expect the same fate as the victim.

Most inhaled poisons interfere in some way with the body's ability to oxygenate the blood. The victim of this type of poisoning, then, is going to suffer low oxygen levels in the blood and needs to be assisted with ventilations. The victim may have ceased to breathe altogether or may need to have a greater volume of oxygen in the lungs. All victims of inhaled poisons need a greater concentration of oxygen in the blood.

The most common sources of inhaled poisons are:

1. chlorine gas — such as that used in swimming pools

2. ammonia fumes — industrial or household

3. carbon monoxide gas — the exhaust fumes from internal combustion engines (cars or other gas-burning engines)

In the case of inhaled poison one should first remove the victim from the source of the poisoning; secondly, activate the EMS system so that adjunctive oxygen equipment can be utilized; and, finally, monitor and assist with ventilation.

INGESTED POISONINGS

There are generally two ways to treat persons who have swallowed poisonous substances. One way is to dilute the poison by having the victim drink water and then cause the person to vomit. The second way to treat poisons which have been swallowed is to dilute the poison and try to keep the victim from vomiting. The decision about which of these methods must be chosen is based on the type of poison swallowed and the level of consciousness of the victim.

When Not to Induce Vomiting

If the victim has swallowed a substance classified as a *corrosive or caustic* agent, vomiting should not be induced. Vomiting might increase the tissue damage done when these substances were swallowed. Inducing vomiting causes more damage as the substance passes back through the stomach, esophagus, pharynx, and mouth.

If the substance swallowed was a *petroleum product or distillate,* vomiting should not be induced. Petroleum products and their distillates have the potential for causing an often fatal form of chemical pneumonia. The risk of these products entering the lungs is too great to justify the limited benefits of *emetics.*

150

Vomiting should not be induced when there is a chance the victim will *aspirate* the contents of the stomach. These situations occur when the victims of poisoning accidents are unconscious, semiconscious, or convulsing. Furthermore, if the patient has a heart condition, ipecac should not be used.

Finally, vomiting should not be induced if you are uncertain of the source of poisoning. There are too many possible negative outcomes from emetics to justify their use in uncertain circumstances.

In summary, *do not induce vomiting* if the following conditions exist:

1. If the ingested substance was a corrosive or caustic agent;

2. If the ingested substance was a petroleum product or distillate;

3. If the victim is unconscious or semiconscious;

4. If you are uncertain of the source of the poisoning.

When to Induce Vomiting

In poisoning emergencies, the rescuer should induce vomiting if the poison control center, a physician or emergency room personnel advise to do so. If no guidance is available from any of these sources, then the decision to induce vomiting must be based on complete knowledge of what was swallowed. If the source of poisoning does not fit into any of the previous four reasons for not inducing vomiting, then the rescuer may proceed.

In order to induce vomiting, the rescuer should administer *syrup of ipecac.* This compound works on *chemical receptors* in the medulla part of the brain. This part of the brain controls many actions which are not under conscious control; one of these reflexes is the vomiting reflex. Vomiting from syrup of ipecac administration is usually quite forceful and efficient in emptying the contents of the stomach. Adults should receive two teaspoons and children over one year of age should receive one teaspoon. Administration of ipecac

should be followed by two eight-ounce glasses of water for adults and one glass for children. This is to insure that there will be something in the stomach to be regurgitated. Vomiting with nothing in the stomach, "dry heaves," can be harmful. If vomiting does not happen within ten to fifteen minutes, one additional dose may be administered.

Once vomiting has occurred, a sample of the vomitus should be saved and transported to the emergency room with the victim for positive identification of the poisonous substance. If a sample of the suspected poisonous agent and its container can be acquired, that too should be brought to the emergency room with the victim. After vomiting is completed, two tablespoons of *activated charcoal* in a glass of water may be given to the patient. This is a rather unappetizing mix, and may require strong persuasion.

Activated charcoal may be administered in some cases when vomiting is not induced to absorb the substance and permit its rapid excretion through the digestive tract. This method of removal is often used when the patient, because of an underlying heart condition, or the risk of aspiration, makes it undesirable to use syrup of ipecac.

CONTACT PLANTS THAT POISON

With the return of spring comes the rich and colorful foliage that makes outdoor living a visual treat. Children often try to turn those visual treats into taste sensations with disastrous results, for some of the beautiful plants festooning our fields, lawns, and homes are poisonous. Children are drawn to the colorful leaves and berries of plants, and a child's curiosity calls for a taste test. The results of this experimental snack may be nausea, convulsions, or coma — even death.

The child's reaction depends on the size and age of the child, toxicity of the plant, and the amount of the plant consumed. Fortunately, the poisons in the plants often taste quite bitter, so the experiment ends quickly. Fortunately, too, the poisons are often very diluted in the plants, so large quantities of them must be consumed to do lasting damage. However, it is still wise to recognize and teach children to recognize the true colors behind the seductive beauty of poisonous plants.

Unfortunately, there is no common characteristic among poisonous plants that makes identification easy — no telltale coloring, no giveaway odor and no given number or pattern of leaves. Some of nature's most delicate and beautiful creations are powerful poisons, from the seasonal poinsettia to the castor bean, bulbs or leaves or berries. The source of the toxicity varies from plant to plant. For example, the rhubarb stalk makes a delicious pie, but its leaf is very poisonous.

The trouble with most plant poisonings is the difficulty of identifying the "guilty" plant. If the exact plant and its toxin are not identified, then the appropriate antidote cannot be identified. Children may not make the association between what was consumed an hour ago and the symptoms now present. Many symptoms of plant poisoning do not appear for several hours or even for one full day after consumption of the plant. In some mushrooms, the onset of symptoms may be delayed even three or four days.

There are, then, two distinct sets of problems in the identification of poisonous plants. The first is the problem of identification of a plant which has been ingested but cannot be identified. In this case, the best course of action is to take a sample of the plant with you to the emergency room for later identification. The second, and perhaps more complex, problem results from delayed reaction to a plant poisoning which may have occurred hours or days previously. In this case, a sample of any vomitus, if present, should be brought to the emergency room with the patient.

Emergency Treatment

Ingestion of poisonous plants is no different from ingestion of any other poison — the best thing you can do is call poison control. If there is no poison control center available to you, the following is the suggested method for handling plant ingestion poisoning:

1. If it has been two hours or less since ingestion of the plant, dilute the contents of the stomach with two glasses of water and induce vomiting.

2. Do not induce vomiting if the poisoning happened more than two hours previously.

3. If you know what has been consumed, bring a sample to the emergency room for positive identification.

4. If the victim regurgitates and you have no sample of the plant, same some of the vomitus for identification.

The accompanying chart identifies common poisonous plants, source of toxin, and symptoms of poisoning.

(The authors gratefully acknowledge the contribution of Kent Perkins of the University of Florida in providing information included on plant poisoning.)

ENVIRONMENTAL POISONINGS

Environmental poisoning may occur as a result of physical contact with an agent which causes irritation to the skin (contact poison) or injected by the bite or sting of an animal or insect (injected poison).

Contact Poisoning

Contact poisoning is by exposure to the oils of plants such as poison ivy, poison oak, and poison sumac. The irritating oils are found on the leaves, stems, roots, and in the smoke of the burning plant. The oils are especially tenacious and thorough washing is needed to get rid of the poison. The oils may remain on clothes, skin, or the coat of pets or other animals. Until the oil is washed off, it may be spread by scratching, rubbing, or any other physical contact.

If the poison is spread through smoke, it is dangerous because it may irritate the lining of the respiratory tract. In children who attempt to ingest these plants, swelling of the mouth and/or pharynx may occur. In these types of poisoning, swelling may reduce the openings of the respiratory passages, making breathing difficult.

The general treatment for contact poisoning is to wash the affected areas thoroughly. Wash all clothing and pets which may have come into contact with the plants. Expose the areas to the air

COMMON PLANTS: TOXINS AND SYMPTOMS

PLANT: COMMON NAME	SOURCE OF TOXIN	SYMPTOMS	WHERE FOUND
Azalea	all parts of plant	nausea, vomiting, difficulty breathing	outdoor shrub
Castor bean	all parts but esp. seeds	thirst, nausea, bloody gastroenteritis with diarrhea, liver/kidney impairment, convulsions	outdoor large annual/costume jewelry (seeds)
Oleander	leaves and branches	severe nausea, irregular heartbeat	outdoor shrub
Poinsetta	leaves, sap, seeds	contact irritant, may cause burning, inflammation and/or blistering of mouth and throat if ingested	indoor/outdoor shrub
Rhubarb	leaf blade	convulsions and possible coma	outdoor vegetable garden
Rubber plant	latex found in leaf and stem	photo dermatitis (extreme sensitivity to sunlight), burning and itching or blistering of skin	indoor/outdoor tree
Dieffenbachia	all parts of plant	burning and itching of mouth and mouth and tongue with possible edema (swelling)	indoor perennial
Mistletoe	berries	cute gastroenteritis and heart failure, copious urination, cramps, vomiting, dilated pupils	outdoor native parasite/indoor cut decoration
Nightshade	all parts	dilated pupils, hot dry flushed skin, convulsions, thready pulse	outdoor native weedy annual
Carolina Jasmine	all parts including flower and nectar	headache, dizziness, dilated pupils, double vision, convulsions, respiratory arrest	outdoor native perennial vine
Barbados Nut	leaves, seeds and sap	burning throat, nausea, abdominal pain, vomiting, labored respiration dehydration	outdoor tree
Pokeweed	all parts, esp. root and purple stem	burning of mouth and cramps, nausea, vomiting, visual disturbance, convulsions, respiratory failure	outdoor native weed
Holly	berries	nausea, vomiting and stupor	outdoor/indoor shrub/tree
Rosary Pea	all parts, esp. seed	gastroenteritis, vomiting, diarrhea, cold sweat, weak fast pulse, cardiac symptoms may not appear for 2 days, extremely toxic- 1 chewed seed may be toxic to adults. If unchewed, seed may pass with no harm	outdoor perennial vine, costume jewelry (seeds)
Elderberry	root, bark, stem and leaves (fruit is edible when cooked and is usually made into jellies and wine)	nausea, vomiting and diarrhea	outdoor shrub
Yellow Allamanda	all parts, esp. sap	vomiting and diarrhea, usually doesn't require treatment	outdoor shrub

and keep them dry. Research seems to indicate that over-the-counter ointments for the treatment of poison oak, ivy, and sumac are probably of little or no benefit.

Injected Poisoning

Poisonous bites and stings come from bees, spiders, marine life, and snakes. Stings from bees produce pain and localized reddening and itching in most people, but may produce exaggerated symptoms in those who are allergic to the venom of the bees. If an individual is bitten or stung repeatedly, or has several bites or stings over a short period of time, enough venom may accumulate to cause a severe reaction. In all of these cases, the reaction is *anaphylactic shock,* which is discussed in Chapter 4.

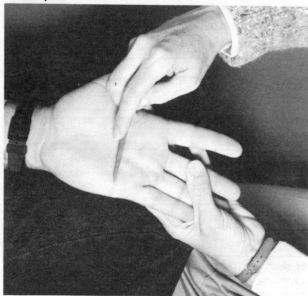

Figure 8-2. *Remove a stinger from the palm with a blade. Scrape the stinger out after carefully looking to see where it is.*

Bee Stings. The stings of bees are of two basic types. First is the sting of bees which have barbed stingers. When these bees sting, the stinger and venom sac remain behind when the bee leaves. The venom sac continues to pulsate, injecting venom into the victim for some time afterward. In this case, the care for bee sting is to remove the stinger and venom sac without squeezing the venom sac. This is accomplished by using a knife blade or other sharp instrument to move the stinger side to side until it is scraped away. Once

the stinger and venom sac are removed, a paste of tap water and meat tenderizer may be applied to the site.

In the case of bees with no barbs on their stingers, the problem is different. Barbless stingers may be withdrawn without disemboweling the bee; thus the bee may repeatedly sting the victim.

Spider Bites. Generally, spider bites result in localized reddening and irritation but little else. There are two types of spider bites, however, which are more serious and occasionally fatal. Different types of spiders produce different types of venom with different effects on the victim. The two types of spiders which produce enough potent venom to be especially serious are the *black widow* and the *brown recluse.*

Recognition of potentially dangerous spiders is an important thing for there is little the rescuer can do once the victim is bitten. From a practical standpoint, the rescuer cannot help beyond thoroughly cleansing the wound, assisting respirations, and transporting the victim to a medical facility. Even in the medical facility, there is no antivenom for black widow and brown recluse bites, so treatment focuses on the management of the resultant symptoms of the bite.

Marine Organisms. Marine organisms can inflict injury through both injection of venom via nematocysts (stinging organs which release venom into the patient's skin) as well as via a direct bite. Commonly, the venom causes a local reaction at the wound site, seen as pain or irritation.

Ordinary rubbing alcohol should be poured over the wound site and left in place for five to ten minutes, inactivating the stingers which have not yet fired. Next, a solution made with water and baking soda should be applied to neutralize the venom. Patients with a more severe reaction to the venom may show signs and symptoms of *analphalaxis.*

Snakebites. Two types of snakes are poisonous in the United States: *pit vipers* and *coral snakes.* Other snakebites of the non-poisonous variety can be treated as any other wound.

Pit vipers (rattlesnakes, cottonmouths and copperheads) are identified by a triangular-shaped head that is wider than the neck, with pits between their eyes and nostrils which appear like an extra set of nostrils. The fangs of the pit viper are exposed during the attack and are used to inject venom into the victim. Coral snakes have bands of red, yellow and black on the body, with black beginning at the nose. The venom of the coral snake is a neurotoxin which causes motor paralysis of the muscles.

The goal of emergency care for snakebite is to reduce the absorption of the toxin at the site. To aid in this, have the victim remain calm and keep movement to a minimum. A broad, constricting band should be placed above the bitten area within thirty minutes of the bite, and the extremity immobilized to minimize movement. The patient should be transported immediately to a hospital. Do not apply ice to the area, as the tissue may be damaged more by the cooling than by the venom. Attempt to identify the snake or bring the dead snake with the victim to the hospital. Attempt to communicate early with the hospital of the patient's impending arrival.

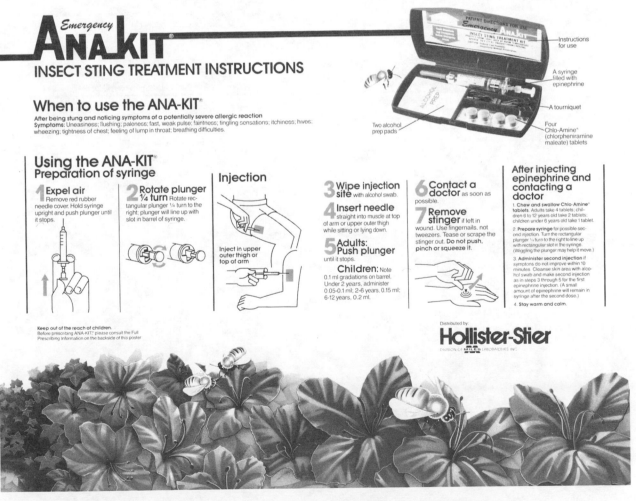

Figure 8-3. *Insect sting treatment kits can protect against severe allergic reactions.*

NOTES

1. Miller and Keane, *Encyclopedia and Dictionary of Medicine, Nursing, and Allied Health.* W. B. Saunders and Company, Philadelphia, 1978, p. 800.

2. Perkins, Kent D. and Willard W. Payne. *Guide to Poisonous and Irritant Plants of Florida.* Published by the University of Florida Extension Service of the Institute of Flood and Agricultural Sciences, # 7-3, 2m-84.

Building Skills: Decisions about Poisoning

Poisoning is a situation where the emergency caregiver can be of particular value to the professional health care provider. The first person to respond to a suspected poisoning—more likely a family member of the victim than a physician or other health care provider—can play a vital role in the outcome of the poisoning. Correct decisions about emergency care made early can be critical. The following skill-building activity is intended to help you improve proficiency in making decisions about how to deal with poisoning.

Directions: For each of the situations given, develop a plan of action. Read the information given, review the appropriate sections of the text and set forth a plan for emergency care.

a.   A neighbor's three -year-old child has apparently eaten some sort of plant or berry. You first learn about this from the child herself and her father. The father is frightened to the point that he is of no help. What you know now is that the child is nauseated, has already vomited, and is having difficulty breathing. She has said something about eating a flower outside, but the information may not be correct. Given her state, her respiration and pulse are okay. What is your plan?

_____

_____

_____

_____

_____

_____

b.   While doing some cleaning in your garage, you were apparently bitten by some type of insect. You have seen lots of different kinds of spiders, but don't know very much about them. The bite on your arm is very painful and reddened, but not bleeding. You have noticed that you are having some difficulty breathing and you are sometimes dizzy. What is your plan?

_____

_____

_____

_____

_____

c.   You are on a backpacking trip and, after hiking through some dense underbrush, one member of the group complains of severe itching on his legs. One of the first times he scratches, he also rubs his eyes (with the same hand). What can you do?

_____

_____

_____

_____

_____

Chapter Nine

Medical Emergencies

In this chapter we change from a strict focus on emergencies associated with accidents to a broader perspective that includes common and not-so-common conditions that may develop suddenly or have a gradual onset, and which may result in emergency situations if not given proper attention early.

First aid for these illnesses and conditions is somewhat different and much more variable than for emergencies discussed earlier. Of course, these situations have the potential to become life-threatening, thus the basic directions for first aid remain in effect. An open airway, breathing, and heartbeat must be established and maintained before attending to any other concerns.

Fainting

Fainting (syncope) is perhaps the most common cause of unconsciousness. The dangers associated with fainting are other injuries from falling and loss of airway. For a victim who feels faint, loss of consciousness may be prevented by lying down with the feet and legs raised 6-12 inches, or by sitting bent over with the head between the knees. Fainting is usually caused by a sudden loss of blood pressure in the brain, so use of gravity to maintain the pressure will usually help prevent loss of consciousness.

In the event the victim loses consciousness, insure an open airway and lay the victim down with feet and legs elevated 6-12 inches. Gentle patting of the hand may help the victim regain consciousness. Seek help if consciousness does not return promptly.

Diabetic Emergencies

Diabetes is a disease in which the body is unable to regulate the amount of sugar (glucose) in the bloodstream. The body must have sugar to function, but the amount present in the bloodstream, for cells to use must be carefully controlled. Too much or too little sugar in the bloodstream causes trouble. Produced by the pancreas, insulin regulates the amount of sugar in the bloodstream. Diabetes mellitus develops when this system for regulating blood sugar goes awry. In nearly all cases, the problem is a lack of insulin.

Individuals who have diabetes are treated by administration of synthetic insulin. Depending on the situation, the insulin may be administered orally (pills) or by injection. In either case, the key to good management is balancing insulin with food that contains sugar. Most individuals with diabetes take insulin on a regular schedule and must adhere to a diet that controls the amount of sugar they consume.

Two different types of problems develop when the system gets out of balance—hyperglycemia (too much sugar in the bloodstream) and hypoglycemia (too little sugar in the bloodstream). Each problem results from the same cause—an imbalance of insulin and food containing sugar.

Hypoglycemia is also known as insulin shock. The victim may develop slurred speech, experience emotional changes, tremors (shaking), feel faint or dizzy. These symptoms usually develop gradually but may overcome the victim very quickly.

Hyperglycemia (too much sugar in the bloodstream) develops when there is an insufficient amount of insulin available to handle blood sugar. As blood sugar rises, the victim may begin to behave as though intoxicated with alcohol. Drowsiness and mental confusion develop and the breath may have a characteristic fruity (acetone) odor. This odor may be confused with that of alcohol unless you are familiar with it.

First Aid. For *hyperglycemia,* the victim must receive medical attention—there are no effective first aid measures for this condition.

For *hypoglycemia*, first aid is to raise blood sugar as soon as possible. Any food that contains sugar can be given to the victim to head off unconsciousness. Early recognition of hypoglycemia is very important, because if the victim becomes unconscious a true medical emergency exists. Transport an unconscious victim with hypoglycemia to a medical facility without delay. Be certain that medical personnel understand that the victim is hypoglycemic so that treatment can begin immediately.

Epilepsy and Other Seizure Disorders

Seizures develop for many reasons. They are characterized by uncontrolled muscle movements, twitching, and drooling. Persons having seizures are not aware of their actions during the seizure. An extremely important thing to remember about seizures is that they are not a disease, but are a sign of disease.

Seizures are among the most upsetting conditions that emergency caregivers encounter. They occur suddenly and without warning or explanation. First aid measures for seizures are summarized below:

1. Remain calm (easier said than done). Seizures are upsetting, particularly to those who have never seen one before. Self-control is essential for first aid.

2. Lower the victim to the floor.

3. Remove anything near the victim which might cause injury—furniture, for example.

4. Position the victim on his or her side to prevent choking. Do not place anything in the victim's mouth.

5. Many victims will appear to have stopped breathing as the seizure ends. Breathing usually begins again shortly. Be certain that the victim has truly stopped breathing before you consider artificial respiration. Cyanosis (blue lips and face) is common as seizures end.

6. Since many seizure disorders are chronic, be sure to ask the victim, or someone familiar with the victim, what should be done following the seizure. Any injuries that occurred during the seizure must be attended to, but in many cases, hospitalization is not needed. If the seizure is a first-time event, the victim should be transported to a health care facility without delay.

Most victims of seizures will have no memory of the event or their behaviors. Be prepared to provide emotional support to such individuals.

Stroke

Stroke is also known as *cerebrovascular accident.* In brief, this condition may develop when the blood supply to the brain is interrupted or damaged. Strokes can strike any part of the brain. Since each part of the brain is responsible for control over specific neurologic body functions, the location and extent of damage from the stroke can be estimated from symptoms.

A basic understanding of how the brain functions will help in recognizing strokes. The brain can be thought of as as divided into halves, each half controlling the opposite side of the body. The left side of the brain controls the right arm, the right leg, and so on. If the left side of the brain is not working properly, the right arm and leg may lose motor function. The right side of the face will also appear to droop because the muscles will not be functional. The right pupil may dilate as well. These are the "classic" symptoms of stroke. Remember that head injuries may produce the same symptoms.

Although the victim of a stroke may not respond verbally and may appear to not comprehend, he or she may be able to hear and understand everything; therefore, discretion should be used in communication.

First Aid. A stroke victim must be transported to a hospital at once. Because stroke may be life-threatening — the part of the brain that is affected may control heartbeat and respiration — pulse and respiration must be monitored. The victim should be positioned with head and shoulders raised slightly. Place the victim on his or her side if there is any danger of choking.

Asthma and Other Respiratory Emergencies

Asthma is a condition in which the lungs react to foreign substances in the air, swell and make the victim short of breath. In extreme cases, the victim's respiratory system may swell to the degree that breathing is all but impossible. Emotional shock may also bring on an "asthma attack."

Allow victims of asthma to assume the position that they find most comfortable. Most find breathing easiest when in a semi-reclining position. Watch for cyanosis—blue color to the lips and face—and be prepared to administer artificial respiration if the victim loses consciousness and stops breathing. Experiencing difficulty breathing often causes panic reactions. Reassurance may be of help in stemming these reactions.

Victims who have chronic asthma may have medicine or sprays with them that will help resolve their symptoms. Seek medical attention for any victim of respiratory attack when there is no history of previous attacks or when the victim loses consciousness.

As reaction to bee stings, food allergies or medicine allergies, some people will develop *ana-phylaxis.* This reaction, characterized by wheez-

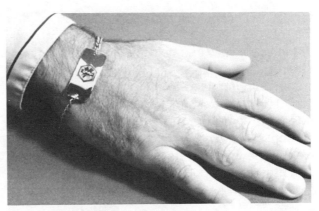

Figure 9-1. *Medical Alert Tag. Found in a variety of shapes and sizes, these tags help alert rescuers to the need for special precaution in administering first aid to a victim. Necklaces and ankle bracelets are also common.*

ing, tightness in the chest, hives and other symptoms, is potentially fatal and must be dealt with immediately. People who have known allergies may wear a medic-alert tag and they may carry a treatment kit with them. (See Figure 9-1.)

Eye Injuries

The eyeball rests in a bony cavity (the orbit) of the skull. The orbit protects the eye from most blunt trauma, while insuring an extensive range of sight. The eye is further protected by the eyelids and eyelashes. It is supplied by numerous blood vessels and nerves and has many muscle attachments.

Injuries to the eye are generally from four sources: (1) blunt trauma to the eye; (2) foreign objects in the eye; (3) penetrating objects to the globe; and (4) burns, either chemical or thermal.

Blunt Trauma. Blunt trauma to the eye may be the result of recreational injuries from balls such as racquetballs, tennis balls or other balls which are smaller than the orbit or may be compressed against the face and forced into contact with the eye. Such injuries in recreational games may be prevented by the use of appropriate protective eyewear.

Three major results from blunt trauma to the eye are swelling within and behind the globe, which causes it to bulge outward; a collection of blood in the anterior chamber of the eye; or a forceful removal of the eyeball from the socket.

If the eye swells and bulges outward, it will need to be moistened, since the ability to tear or blink is usually compromised in this type of injury. The second part of treatment for this type of injury is to protect the eye from further injury. This may be accomplished by the use of a protective eye shield. The injured person should be transported to an emergency room or *ophthalmologist* as soon as possible.

If the colored circle of the eye appears to be darker at the bottom than in the rest of the circle, there may be a collection of blood between the iris and cornea. This is referred to as *hyphema*. This condition requires minimizing movement on the part of the patient and applying a patch to the eye. Again, the patient should be transported to an emergency room or ophthalmologist as soon as possible.

Finally, if the force of the blunt trauma is sufficiently strong, the eyeball may be forcefully removed from its socket. If the eye has been *extruded*, follow this suggested procedure:

1. Cover the eyeball with a moist dressing.
2. Provide a protective covering, such as a cup or commercial eye protection shield.
3. Stabilize the protective cover.

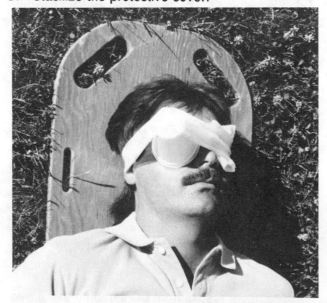

Figure 9-2. *An inverted cup placed over the injured eye and held in place will protect the eye from further injury.*

4. Patch the uninjured eye, remembering to advise the patient of the need to relax and to try not to move the eye.

Foreign Objects in the Eye. Objects may be blown or forced into the eye, remaining on the cornea or inside the lid. If these objects are not lodged in the eye, they may be removed using one of the following techniques.

1. If the matter is under the upper lid, the lid may be gently pulled outward and turned back over a Q-Tip or match stick, thus exposing the underside of the upper lid and making it easy to remove the foreign object.

2. If the object is under the lower lid, this lid may be gently pulled down, exposing the underside of the lower lid. The corner of a dry, clean cloth folded into a triangle may be used to remove these objects.

3. If the object seems to be lodged or adhering to the eyeball, patch both eyes to reduce bilateral movement and transport the person to an ophthalmologist.

Penetrating Injuries to the Eye. Objects that penetrate and/or become embedded in the eye are a special problem. If an object is impaled in the eye, it must be protected from movement since movement may cause further damage to the eye.

Under no circumstances should an impaled object be removed from the eye. Removal of such an object might allow the escape of *vitreous humor* from the eye, endangering sight. Even putting pressure on the globe of the eye with an impaled object in place might cause leakage of fluid from the eye.

The rescuer must use a cup-type bandage to protect the eye and immobilize the impaled object. Remember when treating lacerated wounds of the eyelids or globe of the eye, no direct pressure should be used on the eyeball. *Cover both eyes to prevent movement.*

Burns to the Eye. Burns to the eye may be thermal or chemical in nature. Thermal burns may

162

be caused by the sun, fire, or exposure to intense light such as arc welding or lasers. Thermal burns should be treated by using cool, moist dressings to soothe pain and patches to protect the eyes from further injury. If available, dark-colored patches should be worn to filter light when the injury is sun or light-related.

Chemical burns to the eye must be flushed with clean water immediately and thoroughly. Wash the eye for ten to fifteen minutes, if possible, longer if the burning substance is alkaline. The eye should be flushed from the midline outward so that the matter is not washed from the injured eye to the uninjured eye. If both eyes are burned, then water should be poured over the bridge of the nose so that it drains outward from both eyes.

Injuries to the Ear

The ear is divided into three sections, the outer, middle and inner ear. The outer ear is the portion of the ear most susceptible to soft tissue injury. The *auricle,* or outer appendage of the ear, is subject to damage just as any other soft tissue. The auricle is largely cartilagenous but it is also supplied with blood. Injuries to the auricle may be painful but are not usually life-threatening.

Caution must be used in dealing with ear injuries for two reasons. First, an injury which is the result of force being applied to the outer ear may also cause damage to the middle or inner ear and/or may result in skull fracture, brain damage, or concussion. Second, injuries involving hemorrhage from the ear should be carefully inspected for the presence of cerebrospinal fluid (CSF). Cover and light dressing only.

Nosebleed

Nosebleed is the most common injury to the nose. Nosebleed may be the result of injury to the nose, rupture of small vessels inside the nose, or irritation of the nose.

The victim should be instructed to lean slightly forward so that the blood does not drawn into the throat where it can be swallowed. The nostrils should be pinched together and the victim encouraged to sit quietly. If bleeding persists, gauze may be placed in the nostrils and pressure reapplied, while adding cool compresses to the nose and upper lip. If hemorrhaging continues, the victim should see a physician as the nosebleed could be the result of hypertension, polyps in the nose, vitamin deficiency, or some other medical condition.

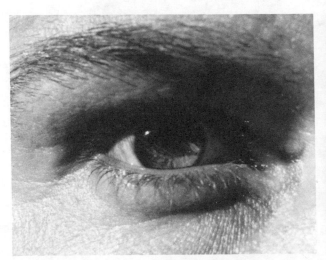

Figure 9-3. *Even though the eye is protected by the orbit (skull bones), eyelid, lashes and tears, it is still very susceptible to injury.*

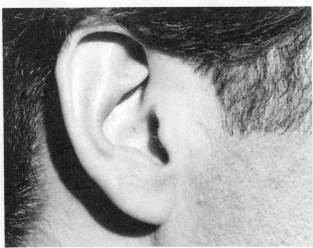

Figure 9-4. *Injuries to the ear include lacerations to the external ear and possibly more serious injury to the sound-conducting mechanisms inside the skull.*

Fingernails and Toenails

Crushing injuries to finger and toe nails often result in bleeding underneath the nail. Since the blood does not have a means of escape, pressure builds under the nail. Pain and throbbing accompanies the pressure. Depending on the injury, the pain can be excruciating. Releasing the pressure under the nail and applying cold will ease the pain and reduce swelling. Application of cold means using ice or cold water; releasing the pressure involves making a small hole in the nail.

There are several choices for procedures for making a hole in the finger or toe nail; two involve emergency caregivers and a third choice is to seek medical attention. For "simple" situations, where there is no doubt about underlying fractures or more serious injuries, the emergency caregiver can make a hole in the nail by using a heated paper clip or a small knife.

The paper clip method: Finger and toe nails are impervious to pain and will melt if subjected to sufficient heat. (The nails are impervious to pain, not the underlying tissues.) Bend a paper clip so that the end of the wire is isolated. It can be heated and applied with gentle force to the injured nail to produce a hole. The trapped blood will be released, and bleeding should cease quickly. Bandage the nail with a sterile dressing.

The small knife method: Sterilize the end of a small knife blade and drill a hole in the nail by turning the knife. The sharper the knife blade, the less painful this procedure will be. Again, bandage the nail with a sterile dressing after the bleeding stops.

Seek medical attention if there is any doubt about the extent or nature of the injury.

ABDOMINAL PAIN

Unexplained severe abdominal pains are often a medical mystery. Experienced physicians often have difficulty coming up with a diagnosis. Even more important, severe abdominal pain is often a sign of illness that is so serious that many individuals will die without treatment. The conclusion that emergency caregivers should draw from these facts is that severe abdominal pain should signal immediate need for medical help. The essential skills that are necessary for the emergency caregiver, therefore, are skills that enable correct assessment of the victim.

Assessment. The abdominal area extends from the bottom of the rib cage to the pubis. To carry out a thorough examination of the abdomen usually requires exposing the skin to the sight and touch of the emergency caregiver.

Try to form a mental picture of the victim's pain as you carry out the examination. Be very systematic, starting in one part of the abdomen and methodically working your way around. Examine the abdominal region first, looking for distension and color alteration (usually redness). Next, lightly feel the abdomen. Does the victim feel pain with even the slightest touch? Does the skin feel hot to the touch? If the victim does not feel pain to light touch palpate the abdomen by pushing your fingers slightly deeper.

Try to determine where the pain is in the abdomen, and when it is worse. Does the pain increase or decrease when you push, as you release pressure, or is it always there? Keep mental note of findings on each of these items and repeat if you cannot arrive at a clear mental picture of the victim's pain.

First Aid. Victims with severe abdominal pain require medical attention. If the victim cannot bear any touching of the abdomen, if the skin is hot to the touch and/or distended, medical attention is needed as soon as possible. The hospital should be warned of the patient's condition before you arrive to allow them to assemble personnel needed for the patient's care. Make certain that the hospital personnel learn of the findings of your examination and the time when it was carried out.

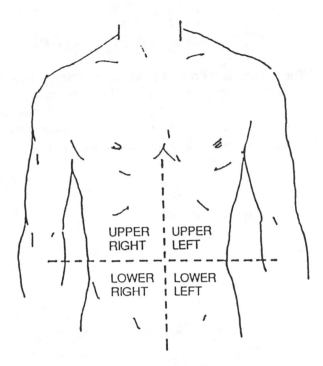

Abdominal quadrants

Do not give patients with abdominal pain anything to eat or drink (surgery is much more dangerous if the patient has eaten or drunk recently). Do not give the patient an enema. Place the patient on his or her back with knees bent to ease the abdominal pain. If nausea or vomiting seem eminent, place the victim on his or her side with knees bent. Monitor the pulse and heartbeat and be prepared to treat for shock.

165

Building Skills

The information presented in this chapter represents a culmination of many of the concepts included in the previous chapters. Like all other emergency situations, a thorough assessment of the problems presented in this chapter forms the basis for actions taken by the emergency caregiver. The activities that follow are intended to help the student in extending skills in assessment and first aid to the types of emergency situations that are common to everyday life.

Directions: The activities that follow are intended to build skills in planning for dealing effectively with common medical emergencies. Read each situation given, find and read the appropriate parts of the text, and develop a plan of action for the emergency caregiver.

1. It is 8:30 A.M. and a 15-year-old student has collapsed on a camping trip. He is conscious but disoriented, very weak and acts "drunk." He denies drinking alcohol, and his friends volunteer the fact that he has diabetes. They don't know if he took his insulin this morning or not.

   a. Is there any other assessment that should be carried out?

   _____

   _____

   b. What should you do or recommend if you decide that the victim is probably in insulin shock? What evidence would support a conclusion of insulin shock?

   _____

   _____

   c. What should you do or recommend if you decide that the victim is hyperglycemic? What evidence would support this conclusion?

   _____

   _____

2. A student suffers an apparent seizure in the cafeteria line. Describe the actions, using the outline below, that should be taken by the emergency caregiver.

   a. Immediate actions

   _____

   _____

   b. Assessment

   _____

   _____

   c. First aid

   _____

   _____

   d. Recommendation for obtaining medical care

   _____

   _____

3. You awake in the middle of the night with abdominal pain. As time passes, the pain increases. What would be the criteria you would use to decide if medical help is needed? For each category of information below, list findings that would lead you toward seeking medical help.

a. pulse and respiration _____

_____

b. temperature _____

_____

c. location of pain _____

_____

d. reaction to touching abdomen _____

_____

e. bowel function (diarrhea or constipation) _____

_____

Chapter Ten

Out-of-Hospital Childbirth

This chapter deals with the special concerns of childbirth occurring outside a medical facility and without medical personnel to oversee the birth. In the greatest number of cases, childbirth will occur naturally and without complications. In a few instances, however, complications may occur and a knowledgeable emergency caregiver can provide first aid. It is the purpose of this chapter to equip the learner with skills necessary to be helpful in either event.

Childbirth in the sterile, controlled atmosphere of today's hospitals is a relatively recent development. In many parts of the world today, and in all societies until the mid-twentieth century, childbirth was considered a routine function not ordinarily requiring specialized medical attention. The emergency caregiver should view childbirth not as an illness but as a natural process. There are dreadful complications associated with childbirth, to be sure, but in the vast majority of cases, the emergency caregiver can act as a helpful stand-in for professional health care providers. Perhaps the most important function of the emergency caregiver is early recognition of potential complications and helping the mother obtain professional medical care.

PREGNANCY

Pregnancy is divided into three periods or trimesters. During each of these trimesters there are a number of developmental activities going on within the mother and the growing fetus. A knowledge of what is happening to the fetus at each stage of pregnancy will aid in understanding the potential dangers of childbirth.

The First Trimester. During the first trimester the fertilized egg is not recognizable as a developing person. After eight weeks, however, the egg is readily identifiable as a growing human and is referred to as a fetus. Early in the first trimester an essential development is the secure attachment of the embryo to the uterine wall. Successful attachment is critical to a fruitful pregnancy. If the fetus does not successfully attach to the uterine wall it will be spontaneously eliminated from the body. This is nature's way of removing a fetus which does not have a chance to develop to maturity and be delivered live.

The Second Trimester. During this phase of development the fetal heart is pumping rapidly and recirculating blood. The developing lungs are collapsed and inactive but formed. The sebacious glands of the skin are producing a slippery coating known as the *vernix caseosa*. The vernix acts as a protective layer between the undeveloped skin and the highly mineralized amniotic fluid. The brain is becoming more convoluted and most major organs will become functional, at least in part. Though the organs look well developed they have not matured enough to function independently. The fetus has no means of regulating its own body temperature and the digestive system cannot function alone. Premature delivery of a fetus at this point would result in death.

The Third Trimester. The final (third) trimester of pregnancy is marked by a slowdown in the rapid development of the fetus. To this point the fetus has grown physically at a rapid rate but this rapid development is slowed to protect the infant from becoming too large to grow and survive within the mother. The fetus becomes less active in the

169

womb but this is because of the lack of available space, not because of the growth slowdown. Sometime during the final month of pregnancy the fetus will assume an upside-down position in preparation for birth. A fetus delivered in the third trimester has a relatively good chance for survival.

LABOR AND DELIVERY

Pre-Labor

Prior to delivery, the mother's body goes through some warm-up activity to prepare for labor. Nature provides exercise for the uterus prior to delivery. The movement of the fetus within the womb causes the uterine muscle to stretch and become more efficient at expelling the fetus at delivery. Late in the third trimester the uterus begins a slow and rhythmic stretching. These "false labor" contractions are known as Braxton-Hicks contractions.

Eventually the fetus will descend in the uterus and begin to pressure the cervix. The combination of pressure on the cervix from the baby's head and the Braxton-Hicks contractions cause the contractions to become stronger and more rhythmic, resulting in labor.

First Stage of Labor

When contractions are no longer Braxton-Hicks contractions but the "real thing," the woman has moved into active labor. The "bloody show," a pink, mucous-like vaginal discharge, is generally a reliable sign that labor has begun. The "bloody show" tells us that the mucous plug which blocks the opening of the cervix is lost. This normally indicates pressure on the cervix from the head of the

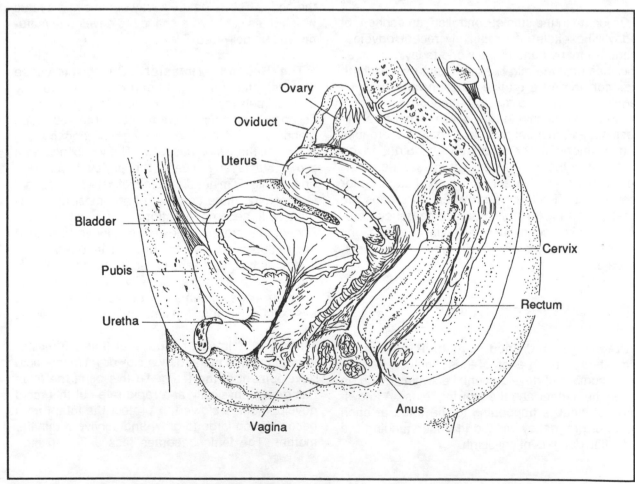

Figure 10-1. *The female reproductive system.*

170

fetus. Sometime after the loss of the mucous plug from the cervix, the **amniotic sac** (bag of waters) will break and the amniotic fluid will be lost. At this point, there will be a gradual dilation of the cervix in preparation for the entry of the fetus into the birth canal.

Second Stage of Labor

When the cervix dilates sufficiently and the fetus enters the birth canal (the vagina), the second stage of labor has begun. During this stage, strong contractions of the uterus will force the baby through the birth canal. This normally takes place in a head-first, face-down position. **Crowning** will indicate the imminent birth of the fetus. Delivery of the fetus indicates the end of the second stage of labor.

Third Stage of Labor

Labor is not finished until the delivery of afterbirth. This usually occurs a few minutes after delivery of the fetus.

ASSISTING DELIVERY

Deciding to Deliver

When a woman goes into labor the first question you must answer is: "How much time do I have before the birth takes place?" To answer this question, first ask about the contractions. Find out how strong the contractions are, how far apart they are and how long they last. In the early stages of labor, contractions last for about one minute, occur every thirty minutes and are something like Braxton-

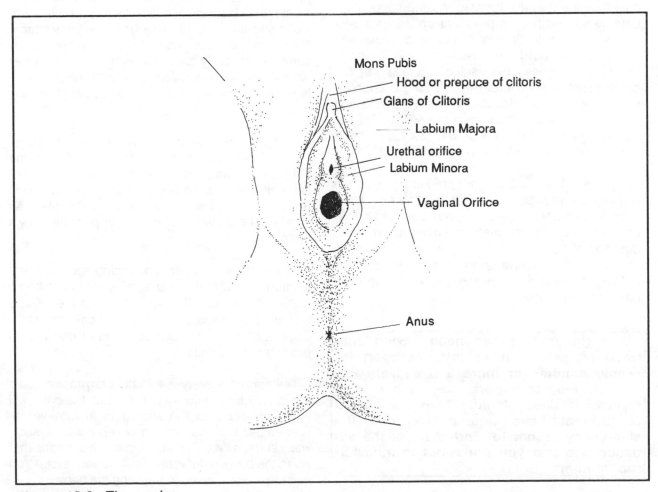

Figure 10-2. *The vagina.*

Mons Pubis
Hood or prepuce of clitoris
Glans of Clitoris
Labium Majora
Urethal orifice
Labium Minora
Vaginal Orifice
Anus

Hicks contractions in strength. As labor progresses contractions get stronger, come closer together and last longer.

Next find out which pregnancy this is for the woman. Labor for a first pregnancy may last fourteen to sixteen hours. Subsequent pregnancies may not have labor periods that last as long. As a result of previous pregnancies, the uterus becomes stronger and more efficient in the birth process. In a second or third pregnancy, labor may last six to eight hours. These are only generalizations, however. The length of labor is unpredictable.

Once you have an idea of the amount of time left based on information about contractions, you should check further. In a situation of emergency childbirth it is not surprising to find that an individual may over- or underestimate time based on the emotion of the situation. Next, ask the woman if she has to move her bowels. A positive response may indicate that the baby is moving through the birth canal and putting pressure on the gastro-intestinal tract resulting in a feeling of a need to defecate. Do not let the woman go to the bathroom. If she does, the vaginal opening may become contaminated and the straining is counterproductive at this point of delivery. Finally, look at the vaginal opening to check for crowning. Do this without touching the vaginal area as you must be careful not to contaminate the delivery field.

If you find there is sufficient time to transport the woman to a medical facility for the delivery, this is your first choice. If there is not enough time to transport the woman, then you must assist in the delivery of the baby. Under no circumstances should the caregiver attempt to delay the birth by holding the mother's legs together or through any other artificial means.

> **If the mother has been having contractions two to three minutes apart for twenty minutes or more and delivery has not started, transport the mother to a medical facility. If more than one person is present have one person call the emergency room to alert them of the situation and that you are about to transport the mother.**

Normal Delivery

Everything near the delivery must be as sterile or clean as possible. Have the mother lie on a clean sheet. Pick up the sheet at her buttocks, raising her a few inches. Place clean towels or a small pillow under the buttocks so they are raised two or three inches. Drape the mother's stomach with a clean sheet and place sterile (or as clean as you can find) towels under the opening of the vagina.

Soon the baby should crown. When crowning occurs, gentle counterpressure should be applied to the top of the baby's head. This is necessary to keep the baby from being born in an explosive fashion. If the baby moves too fast through the vaginal opening, the sudden loss of pressure can result in the tearing of membranes in the baby's head, resulting in death.

If the baby crowns and the amniotic sac has not ruptured, you should rupture it. Again, using the most sterile instrument available, puncture the amniotic sac and push it away from the baby's face. Remember that the baby's head is the largest circumference body part; therefore, it will deliver slowly. As the shoulders and then the hips and legs are delivered the birth becomes progressively more rapid.

As the baby's head is delivered, you must remove blood, mucous and amniotic fluid from the baby's nose and mouth. A bulb syringe is especially efficient, but if one is not handy, you can wipe the mouth and nose with a sterile (clean) cloth. As soon as the airway is cleared, support the baby's head.

The infant should begin breathing spontaneously shortly after birth. If breathing does not begin within 30 seconds, flip the bottoms of the infant's feet with your fingers. If respiration does not start, begin artificial respiration at a rate of one breath every three seconds.

The normal delivery is with the baby facing down but shortly after delivery of the head, the baby will begin to rotate as the shoulders are delivered. Remember that the fetus is covered with a slick, waxy substance called the vernix. This means that when the baby is delivered it will be very slick. You must exercise caution in handling the baby.

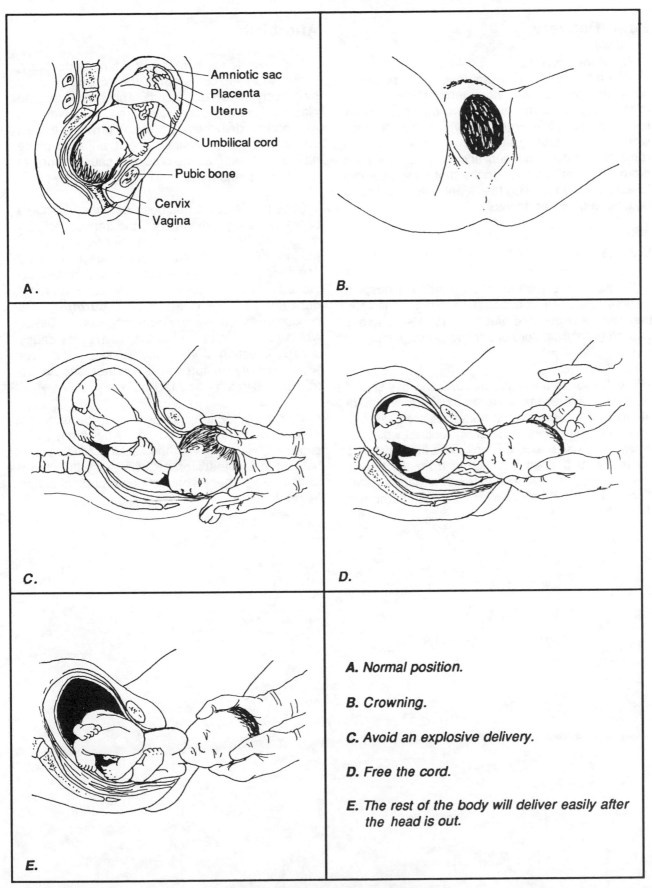

A. Normal position.

B. Crowning.

C. Avoid an explosive delivery.

D. Free the cord.

E. The rest of the body will deliver easily after the head is out.

Figure 10-3. *Steps in Delivery.*

173

Post Delivery

Once the baby has been delivered, it should be wrapped in a blanket. Remember , the baby has no means of regulating body temperature, so you must keep it from losing critical core body temperature. Place the baby on the mother's stomach in a slightly head-down position so that remaining blood, mucous and amniotic fluid will drain. Also, in this position the mother will be able to assist you in holding the infant, allowing you to be free to do other things.

Cutting the Cord

Transport the mother and infant to a hospital without delay. If transportation is not immediate, then the umbilical cord must be cut. Also, *if at any time the umbilical cord ceases to pulse, it must be cut.*

In order to cut the umbilical cord, two ties should be made on the cord. Use the most sterile materials available. If no sterile materials are available, take the time to boil or soak in alcohol whatever you plan to use to cut the cord. The first tie should be made at a point ten inches from the baby's navel and one tie five inches from the baby's navel. The cord should be cut midway between the two ties.

Afterbirth

About five to ten minutes after birth of the baby, some blood will come out of the vagina, followed by delivery of part of the cord. This signals that the placenta has separated from the uterine wall and will soon be delivered. Do not do anything to help delivery of the placenta since it will take place naturally. Pulling on the cord may cause tearing of the placenta and result in serious problems.

Once the placenta has been delivered, it should be saved along with the cord and transported with the mother to the hospital. At the hospital, the afterbirth will be examined to determine if it delivered completely. Some of the afterbirth may remain attached to the uterus. If this is the case, a procedure known as a **dilation and curettage** is necessary to remove any remaining tissue. Tissue which remains attached to the uterus may cause serious infection. If the placenta does not deliver within twenty minutes, the mother should be transported to a medical facility.

After the afterbirth has delivered, the mother's lower abdomen should be gently but firmly massaged. This, along with the sucking action of the baby at the mother's breast, will cause the uterus to contract. These contractions reduce bleeding from the uterus.

OBSTETRIC EMERGENCIES

At various stages of pregnancy there are risks to the health of both the mother and fetus. *In all cases, a physician's help should be sought if at all possible.* The following are the most frequently occurring medical emergencies associated with childbirth.

Toxemia

Toxemia develops in many women during pregnancy. In this condition, the woman begins to gain weight rapidly and retain a great deal of fluids. A result of the fluid retention is that pressure in the arteries is elevated. Because of elevated arterial pressure, arterioles may spasm, which decreases the kidneys' ability to function properly.

This is dangerous because during normal pregnancy the kidneys need to function at a higher rate than normal due to the demands placed by the developing fetus. Toxemia patients should restrict salt intake but increase water intake. This restriction should be within reason and only under the supervision of a physician, as any dietary changes in the mother affect the fetus.

Breech Birth

Occasionally a baby will be born in the breech position. In this instance, the baby is descending the birth canal bottom-first instead of head-first as is normal. Breech refers to the buttocks, and in breech birth the buttocks are the presenting part.

In a breech birth, delivery is the same as for normal presentations except the buttocks and legs come out first and must be supported. Remember that the head is the largest circumference of any body part and will probably deliver more slowly in breech presentation.

If the body delivers but the baby's head is not out three minutes after the rest of the body, or if any other body part presents (an arm or leg, for example), then transportation should be immediate.

Building Skills

The most formidable challenge for the emergency caregiver in dealing with emergency childbirth is deciding whether sufficient time exists before delivery to safely transport the expectant mother to a hospital or medical center. Fortunately, there are guidelines for making such decisions. The activities that follow are intended to help in summarizing and focusing the materials presented in the chapter in terms of making decisions about emergency childbirth.

Chapter Ten: Building Skills

Name_____

Directions: The items listed below outline the logical decision-making process for emergency child-birth. Each item draws on material presented in various parts of the chapter. Find and carefully read the appropriate parts of the chapter for each item, then write out brief statements summarizing the material.

1. How much time? Briefly describe how information provided by each of the following contributes to estimation of the time until delivery.

   a. Number of previous deliveries/pregnancies

     _____

     _____

     _____

   b. Duration of labor

     _____

     _____

     _____

   c. Time between contractions

     _____

     _____

     _____

   d. Bag of waters broken and when

     _____

     _____

     _____

   e. Mother feels strain and need to defecate

     _____

     _____

     _____

   f. Crowning

     _____

     _____

     _____

2. When to transport? Looking over your answers in No. 1:

    a. Which provides the best information about the advisability of transporting a woman in labor?

    _____

    _____

    _____

    b. Are there other factors that should be included in deciding about transport?

    _____

    _____

    _____

3. When is help needed? Describe the conditions under which emergency medical assistance *must* be obtained without delay because of the following:

    a. Bleeding

    _____

    _____

    _____

    b. Presentation of an arm or leg

    _____

    _____

    _____

    c. Labor that does not progress

    _____

    _____

    _____

Chapter Eleven

Crisis Intervention

Rather than focusing on providing first aid to maintain physical health, this chapter will be primarily concerned with interactions between physical and emotional aspects of health. The chapter begins by considering the general principles of first aid in situations in which extreme emotional reactions are possible. The sections that follow will apply emergency care principles to anxiety, threatened suicide, alcohol intoxication and untoward effects of drugs.

EMOTIONAL TRAUMA

All emergency situations have emotional impact. However, emergency situations and the emotional makeup of people vary considerably, which makes it difficult to predict emotional responses. The emergency caregiver should know that strong emotional responses are likely to develop in accident victims, family members and onlookers, and should be prepared to provide emotional first aid as well as help for physical injuries.

In dealing with emotions, the most fundamental principle to remember in emergency care is that reactions in victims and others are a natural and reasonable result of the situation. Secondly, being in a state of emotional distress hinders effective communication because all thoughts and feelings are distorted. Consequently, the usual paths of communication between rescuer and others may not function as expected under normal circumstances. Victims and witnesses may not be able to understand questions and may misinterpret actions of the rescuer. They may become violent and abusive, or inappropriately withdrawn.

Being emotionally upset means:
Distortion of thoughts
Extreme reactions

First Aid

—Professional manner
—Listening
—Effective Communication
—Protect Against Unexpected Changes

The most basic, and perhaps the most valuable, first aid measures that can be rendered to the emotionally upset are a professional manner, careful listening, and effective communication.

A professional manner can be defined as one of compassionate objectivity. This means acting with compassion for the victim's discomfort without becoming emotionally involved to the extent that clear thinking is impaired. A victim whose injuries are upsetting to him/herself and others will almost certainly be upset further if the emergency caregiver is upset and unable to render aid objectively. In addition, the judgment of the caregiver will surely be distorted if control over emotions is lost. Maintaining compassionate objectivity is sometimes easier said than done, to be sure, but the emergency caregiver must make every effort to maintain control.

Listening is the most fundamental part of communication. Listen to the concerns and anxieties of the victim and others. For victims and others, an attentive listener offers reassurance and often has a calming effect.

People who are emotionally upset are often further upset when any unexpected change occurs, however minute. Explaining clearly and carefully all first aid procedures before carrying them out is helpful in reducing unexpected change.

Finally, guard against making judgments about the future. Avoid statements such as "everything will be okay" unless you are absolutely certain that it is so. Neutral statements that describe what is being done for the injured—"we're going to splint this leg"—and conversation about everyday topics that involve the victim (if possible) and others often help to reduce tension.

ANXIETY

Anxiety is a term that describes different types of thoughts and feelings common to emergency situations. As used here, anxiety is a disturbance of the emotions associated with reactions to a specific stressful accident or incident. It is important to realize that anxiety can be displayed in a number of ways and has a variety of symptoms. (See Figure 11-1.)

Emotional responses from anxiety range from little or none to moderate to blind panic. Balance between the seriousness of the situation and emotional reactions is the hallmark of "normal" anxiety. The emergency caregiver should be particularly attentive when there is an imbalance between the situation and the emotional response displayed. Little or no emotional response shown when a situation would ordinarily elicit a severe response, such as sudden death of an infant, may be a very important sign of severe anxiety that may be expressed later. The apparent "self-control" shown in this type of response may mask serious emotional reactions that require treatment. Anxiety displayed as panic is usually apparent and requires immediate management.

Once again, the key question for the emergency caregiver is whether the anxiety shown matches the situation. Special care must be given to situations where anxiety and the situation do not match.

The accident victim, friend or relative, or bystander suffering from anxiety can benefit from attention from the emergency caregiver. A few simple guidelines for emergency caregiving behavior will be very helpful in all but the most extreme cases—such as threatened suicide and panic.

First, identify yourself and take a few minutes to be sure the victim is well-oriented to his or her surroundings. For example, after identifying yourself, explain your first aid plans. Ask if there is anyone— family members, for example—who should be notified about the accident.

Second, listen to what the victim has to say and take the situation seriously in all cases. Listen to the fears and anticipation of the victim without judgment. Accept what the victim says without taking anything personally. Carefully correct misinterpretations of the situation. Do not rush or try to force decisions on an emotionally unstable person—this only exaggerates the problem.

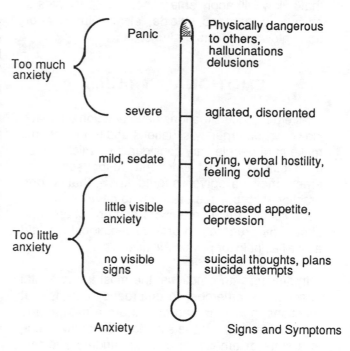

Figure 11-1. *Anxiety is displayed in a number of ways, ranging from panic to no visible signs at all. Emergency caregivers should look for balance between the situation and the behavior seen.* Adapted from Rosa-Grippa, MK. Psychiatric Emergencies. *In the Practice of Emergency Care,* second edition. New York, Lippincott, 1984.

180

Third, remove the victim from an environment where anxiety is likely to be heightened. If possible, get the victim away from the scene to a calm environment where hot drinks and food can be obtained. Do not force people away from an accident scene, however, because for some not knowing about the status of a situation causes additional anxiety.

Panic. When panic strikes and people lose all control, direct intervention is needed. Above all, remain calm yourself. Do not try to restrain any adult alone. Continue to talk soothingly. Continue to try to engage the individual in conversation.

Hyperventilation. Hyperventilation is uncontrolled, prolonged, rapid breathing. This condition occurs when there is sufficient carbon dioxide in the bloodstream—another term for hyperventilation is "O_2 (oxygen) poisoning." The hyperventilating victim may complain of feeling increasingly anxious, lightheaded or dizzy. Anxiety is a common cause of hyperventilation. Rebreathing his or her own exhaled air increases the oxygen in the lungs and will restore normal respirations.

First Aid for Hyperventilation. Explain what you are going to do clearly and carefully first. Then place a paper bag over the victim's nose and mouth and have the victim breathe with the paper bag in place. Regular breathing should return after a few minutes.

SIDS

Sudden Infant Death Syndrome (SIDS) is fortunately a rare occurrence. Infants die unexpectedly, often in the early morning hours. The impact of SIDS is devastating, and is not limited to the family. Emergency caregivers report that SIDS is a very emotionally wrenching experience for them too.

Even though there are no confirmed causes of SIDS, people naturally look for a reason for these catastrophic events. In their state of emotional

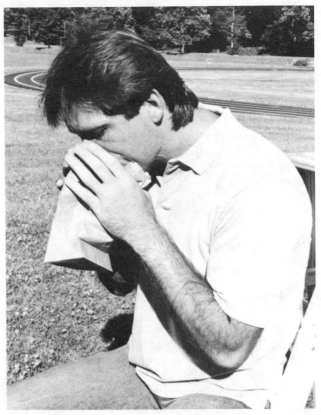

Figure 11-2. *Use a paper bag for treatment of hyperventilation*

distress, even casual questions asked of the parents are usually interpreted as threatening. What the parents need is reassurance that their actions did *not* cause the death of their baby.

Emergency care for SIDS begins with the ABCs. Arrange for assistance as soon as possible and continue with rescue attempts until relieved. Approach the parents with a *nonjudgmental attitude,* aware of their emotionally distressed state.

SEXUAL ASSAULT

Emergency care for victims of sexual assault must be carried out in accordance with first aid principles *and* local legal procedures. When they become victims of assault of a sexual nature, the reactions of human beings vary widely. Some people become violent while others become withdrawn. The emergency caregiver must accomplish three primary goals in providing aid to these victims:

1. Provide first aid for injuries.

2. Take steps to preserve legal evidence of the crime.

3. Provide emotional support.

Preserving legal evidence of the crime includes urging the victim to go to a hospital immediately without doing anything to change his or her condition. Urge the victim to avoid washing, changing clothes, drinking, eating, using the bathroom, or in anyway disturbing evidence. Warn the hospital that a victim of sexual assault is being brought in so necessary preparation for treatment can be made. Most hospitals are equipped and trained to deal effectively with victims of sexual assault and will be able to carry out the examination and treatment while preserving evidence of the crime.

Emotional support is crucial for victims of sexual assault. Long-term therapy may be needed. Assure the victim that he or she is safe and that you will not allow any further harm to come to him/her. Carefully explain the need for preserving evidence and try to persuade the victim to actively help in the process.

THREATENED SUICIDE

A person threatening suicide is essentially upset. Furthermore, the person's behavior is likely to be unpredictable. The emergency caregiver encountering a suicide threat should first arrange for help in dealing with the situation. Law enforcement personnel should be contacted and apprised of the situation without delay.

In dealing with the individual threatening suicide, first establish that there are no weapons involved that could injure others. Move away if the individual has a weapon or if moving away is not possible, initiate a conversation in an attempt to distract the individual.

The key elements to preventing suicide are effective communication and ambivalence. Effective communication demonstrates the value of living while acknowledging the psychic pain of the victim ("Are you thinking of killing yourself?"). Ambivalence means that the victim has not firmly decided on suicide and may be persuaded to try to live (Victim: "I can't see any reason to go on.").

Begin conversations with victims by encouraging them to describe their family, friends and other connections with life. Don't try to make the victim feel guilt about ending his/her life ("What will all these people do?"). Rather, ask how you can help. Maintain the conversation until professional help can be obtained. Once again, communication is the key.

ABUSE OF DRUGS AND ALCOHOL

Drug and alcohol abuse are, unfortunately, very common in our society. Accidents involving substance abuse place the emergency caregiver in a slightly different position from other emotional health emergencies because the effects of substance abuse may exert strong influence on perceptions of the abuser. Behavior of people under the influence of drugs and/or alcohol is very likely to be distorted, making it difficult to obtain reliable information. In addition, and of critical importance, the drug or alcohol abuser may develop physical health problems in addition to the distortion of emotions, due to properties of the substance abused. Depressants such as alcohol can, in sufficient doses, cause cessation of breathing. Stimulants such a cocaine can result in the same outcome. The emergency caregiver must cope with physical injuries in light of alterations in body functions that result from substance abuse.

Alcohol Intoxication

The body is able to process alcohol at a fixed rate. When intake of alcohol exceeds this rate, intoxication occurs. As the dose of alcohol increases, the depression of brain activity progresses. In low to moderate doses, effects include decreased inhibitions and feelings of warmth. In higher doses muscle coordination becomes impaired causing unsteadiness in walking. In very high doses bodily functions are grossly impaired and breathing may cease. Nausea and vomiting may occur with all levels of intoxication.

First Aid. There is no way to speed up the body's rate of processing alcohol. Time is the only cure for alcohol intoxication. Mild stimulants such as coffee (with caffeine) may enhance alertness, but intoxication will continue until the alcohol has been metabolized. Perhaps the most important action to be taken with intoxicated people is to prevent accidents by stopping them from attempting to drive automobiles or operate machinery. Antacids may ease nausea and fruit juices may also be of help in recovering from alcohol intoxication, but time is the primary healer.

Alcohol intoxication becomes acute when the individual can no longer care for him/herself. At sufficient levels of intoxication, breathing becomes labored and respirations may cease. Such individuals may aspirate vomitus and choke if not attended to properly. Allow intoxicated individuals to rest without interference so long as breathing is stable and nausea is not evident. If semiconscious or unconscious, place the victim on his/her side. If breathing seems labored and irregular, see that the individual receives medical attention without delay.

Substance Abuse

Drugs are substances that produce effects on the mind, body, or both. (Alcohol is a drug, but is covered separately because of the prevalence of "accepted" use in society.) Abuse of drugs, as far as the emergency caregiver should be concerned, can be considered a special category of poisoning. People in our society have been known to abuse a wide variety of substances including prescription drugs, over-the-counter medicines, household or industrial cleaning agents, and mood-modifying street drugs. For the purposes of rendering first aid, substance abuse can be divided into three broad categories based on the type of drug(s) involved: stimulants, depressants and hallucinogens.

Stimulants. Stimulants are very common—caffeine found in coffee and many soft drinks is a stimulant. Cocaine, another stimulant, is one of the most commonly abused drugs. When under their effects, users of stimulants are commonly overly excited, restless, and irritable. Overdose of such substances may produce psychological as well as physical symptoms including suspiciousness and paranoia, dizziness, flushed skin, vomiting and convulsions. Respiratory failure may also occur.

Depressants. Depressants include a wide variety of illegal, prescription and over-the-counter drugs. The principal action of all these drugs, however, is to slow body functions. For the emergency caregiver, respirations should be carefully assessed and monitored. Respirations may cease altogether given sufficient dosage.

Hallucinogens. Hallucinogenic agents have the ability to alter the perceptions of all of the user's senses. Effects range widely from extreme pleasure to horror, and are generally unpredictable. Importantly, those under the influence of hallucinogenic substances may have altered perceptions such that they may interpret offers of help as threats. Be careful not to touch the person since this may result in panic.

First Aid for Substance Abuse. Procedures rendering aid to victims under the influence of drugs or alcohol are basically the same as those for any other injured individual. First things first: insure an open airway, check the pulse, and attend to physical injuries. Monitor respiration and pulse carefully, since effects of drugs (depressants particularly) are likely to become apparent in disturbed breathing and irregular or speeded heartbeats. Concerning first aid for symptoms of substance abuse, the nature of the substance abused dictates actions of the emergency caregiver.

1. If the victim is semiconscious or unconscious, position the victim on his/her side to prevent choking.

2. Arrange for medical help as soon as possible. Obtain advice on first aid that can be carried out immediately.

3. Attempt to find out what was taken, when and in what dose.

4. Collect and save all evidence of the substance abused. Bottles, vomitus and any other clues

WHEN THE HELPERS NEED HELP

After a serious accident, the victims aren't always the only ones who feel pain. The emergency caregivers can hurt too. They often become emotionally attached to the victims they help and feel sorry for them and their family members. Although the victims usually are strangers, it's common for care givers to feel compassion for them and even follow their recovery process for days—sometimes weeks—after the disaster.

Doctors, nurses and other health professionals who see the injured every day, though, are trained to maintain a professional detachment. Usually their involvement with patients is short-term. They learn to view the next person to come through the emergency room door as a human organism who needs medical care, and they use their knowledge and skills to provide that care. They're discouraged from getting too close to a patient's case and becoming too involved emotionally.

So how do first-aid givers who have *not* had detachment training keep a professional distance between themselves and the people they treat? It's easier to do if the victims are all strangers. But if the victims are friends or acquaintances—people you care about and love—staying detached after a disaster is nearly impossible.

That's what the crew of AirCare, the helicopter ambulance program at North Carolina Baptist Hospital in Winston-Salem, learned first-hand. In September 1986, their new helicopter crashed in the hills of southwestern Virginia, killing the two flight nurses and pilot aboard. The crash shocked the other crew members, forcing them to cope with the tragic loss of three of their best friends.

"Suddenly, you have this terrible grief reaction," says Dr. Daniel G. Sayers, medical director of AirCare. "You've got tears in your eyes and your heart sinks and your belly feels like it's got lead in it. And there's only about one thing to do in that situation and that is to grab hold of somebody and hug them. A lot of times, all it does is soothe you, I think. It isn't therapy, exactly; it's just a sort of a port in a storm, a rock to cling to."

Courtesy Tyler Cox

These reactions are typical of the way people feel after a tragedy. Second thoughts and doubts about the accident and emergency care are also common. Emergency caregivers are people first, rescuers second. Emotional upset following serious accidents is normal and reasonable and time is the only cure. When the upset feelings do not resolve or if they are so intense that effectiveness is jeopardized, professional help should be sought.

to the identity of the substance should be saved and given to those rendering medical help.

5. Maintain a calm environment around the individual and continually monitor his/her behavior. Some victims may be aided by reassuring conversation ("talking down') but this may also be ineffective. Victims using PCP (phencyclidine) do not ordinarily respond well to conversation and may become more agitated. Provide a quiet, nonstimulating environment for these individuals.

6. Do not attempt to restrain a substance abuse victim without help.

SUMMARY

The most important point to remember from this chapter is that first aid for all injuries is not complete without attention to emotional reactions. For those injured, their relatives and friends, and even bystanders, accidents are traumatic events. The emergency caregiver needs to insure that such emotions are acknowledged and that those with serious reactions are provided access to care. Individuals under the influence of drugs and alcohol also require special attention. Given the alteration of perceptions that often accompanies substance abuse, special attention to clear communication and understanding is needed. Judging and blaming the individual for his or her actions is not the role of the emergency caregiver!

FURTHER READING

Rose-Grippa, M.K. Psychiatric Emergencies. IN J.H. Cosgriff and D.L. Anderson, eds. *The Practice of Emergency Care,* 2nd ed. New York, Lippincott, 1984.

Halpern, J.S. Care of the Poisoned or Overdosed Patient. IN J. H. Cosgriff and D.L. Anderson, eds. *The Practice of Emergency Care,* 2nd ed. New York, Lippincott, 1984.

BUILDING SKILLS

Under emotional stress, human beings sometimes lose control of their faculties. Ordinarily rational, reasonable people can become abusive or totally withdrawn. The emergency caregiver should be able to recognize potentially stressful situations and anticipate unusual behavior. Drug abuse may also produce unexpected behavior. As in the case of emotionally stressful situations, the emergency caregiver should be prepared to provide first aid for the mind of the drug abuser as well as the body.

Name_____

Directions: For each situation described below, develop a plan of action for the emergency caregiver. The plan should include first aid for physical as well as emotional problems suffered by the victim.

a. Walking home one evening, you become involved with a case of sexual assault. A young women has apparently been abducted, raped, beaten and left in a city park. When you arrive, several people are trying to comfort the young woman, but no one has begun any first aid. Outline the steps you would take in this situation.

_____

_____

_____

_____

b. You are at a party with a large number of people. A twenty-one-year-old man has apparently passed out, presumably from drinking too much. Knowing that you have had some first aid training, your friends ask you to make sure he's okay. Your ABC survey shows slowed respiration and heartbeat, pale skin and only brief semiconsciousness after pinching one of his thumbs. As you talk to his friends, the man's breathing starts to become labored and noticeably slowed. The friends mention something about his taking "downers" earlier in the evening. What is your plan?

_____

_____

_____

_____

EPILOGUE

This text is about emergency care, providing first aid to those who have become injured or ill. There is always need for individuals with training in first aid, given the unpredictable nature of accidents and illnesses. Remember the first rule of medical care, for it is particularly applicable to emergency caregivers: **Do no harm.**

A careful and thorough assessment of victims is the best means to prevent doing harm. **Look** at the victim in the context of the accident or illness. **Listen** to what the victim and witnesses report. **Assess** the victim's injuries carefully. In today's society, with our ever-expanding ability to quickly transport professional rescue personnel to where they are needed, perhaps the best advice for the emergency caregiver is to provide immediate care needed and make certain that no further harm comes to the victim while professional rescuers are en route.

EXERCISES FOR REVIEW   Name_____

Directions: The following simulated accident situations have been developed to help the student think about how the topics presented in the text fit together, and how they might be applied in providing emergency care. For each scenario, carry out any procedures requested, render any additional first aid needed, and note the type of additional help needed, if any. In addition, write down a record of your actions including the following:

a. Injury type(s) and location(s). *Example:* laceration above right eyebrow with possible internal head injury

b. Immediate first aid rendered. *Example:* gentle, direct pressure used to control bleeding, dressing and bandage applied.

c. Other information needed by medical professionals. *Example:* witnesses report possible loss of consciousness of 2-3 minutes, victim disoriented and nauseated.

d. Victim report of the mechanism of injury (use the victim's exact words whenever possible)

1. The victim is a male in his mid-fifties. You find him in an office building, unconscious but breathing. He gives no response, despite repeated attempts to arouse him. As you carry out a head-to-toe survey, you note a sickly, sweet odor on his breath.

a. Injury type(s) and location(s)   _____

_____

_____

_____

b. Immediate first aid rendered   _____

_____

_____

_____

c. Other information needed by medical professionals   _____

_____

_____

_____

_____

2. The victim is a fourteen-year-old female, who has fallen and hit her head while roller skating. You find her lying on her back. She denies losing consciousness, but is nauseated. What other information do you need from the victim? What first aid should be provided immediately?

a. Injury type(s) and location(s) _____
_____
_____

b. Immediate first aid rendered _____
_____
_____

c. Other information needed by medical professionals _____
_____
_____

d. Victim report of the accident, how the injury occurred, how she feels now and any other information. _____
_____
_____

3. As a result of an auto accident, this victim has sustained a serious head injury. He has a large bruise on his forehead and a deep laceration, beginning above the left eyebrow and extending down through the eyelid. The victim is conscious but disoriented and smells of alcohol.

a. Injury type(s) and location(s) _____
_____
_____

b. Immediate first aid rendered _____
_____
_____

c. Other information needed by medical professionals _____
_____
_____

d. Victim report of the accident, how the injury occurred, how she feels now and any other information. _____
_____
_____

4. This victim wrecked on a motorcycle. ABC and head-to-toe surveys reveal the following: rapid, shallow respiration; tingling in the arms and legs; tenderness on the left side of the rib cage. The victim appears to be gagging, but there is no blood visible.

a. Injury type(s) and location(s)   _____

_____

_____

b. Immediate first aid rendered   _____

_____

_____

c. Other information needed by medical professionals   _____

_____

_____

d. Victim report of the accident, how the injury occurred, how she feels now and any other information.   _____

_____

_____

5. This victim is a woman in her twenties who has fallen while horseback riding. She was alone when the accident happened, and the horse may have rolled over her. She cannot remember and is very short of breath. In your surveys you find that she appears to have a right clavicle injury and her ribs are injured on both sides of the sternum. You notice a slight cavity in her rib cage on the opposite side from the clavicle when she inhales.

a. Injury type(s) and location(s)   _____

_____

_____

b. Immediate first aid rendered   _____

_____

_____

c. Other information needed by medical professionals   _____

_____

_____

d. Victim report of the accident, how the injury occurred, how she feels now and any other information.   _____

_____

_____

6. An eight-year-old boy has been hit by a car while riding his bicycle. You find breathing and heartbeat, numerous abrasions, and tenderness of the left arm and shoulder. The victim is responsive and talkative. On more careful examination, you find what appears to be knotted muscles just above the left elbow.

a. Injury type(s) and location(s) _____

_____

_____

b. Immediate first aid rendered _____

_____

_____

c. Other information needed by medical professionals _____

_____

_____

d.   Victim report of the accident, how the injury occurred, how she feels now and any other information. _____

_____

_____

7. This victim tells you that his "trick" shoulder has popped out. He goes on to say that he has very little feeling in his arm and hand. Examination of the limb shows a bluish color and no pulse.

a. Injury type(s) and location(s) _____

_____

_____

b. Immediate first aid rendered _____

_____

_____

_____

c. Other information needed by medical professionals _____

_____

_____

d.   Victim report of the accident, how the injury occurred, how she feels now and any other information. _____

_____

_____

Name_____

8. This victim was a loser in a knife fight. The handle is clearly visible between the fifth and sixth ribs on the right side. The victim is lying on his back, is short of breath and showing signs of shock. He has frothy, bright red blood in his mouth.

a. Injury type(s) and location(s) _____

_____

_____

b. Immediate first aid rendered _____

_____

_____

c. Other information needed by medical professionals _____

_____

_____

d. Victim report of the accident, how the injury occurred, how she feels now and any other information. _____

_____

_____

9. A football accident has left this victim with an open fracture of both the radius and ulna of the right arm.

a. Injury type(s) and location(s) _____

_____

_____

b. Immediate first aid rendered _____

_____

_____

c. Other information needed by medical professionals _____

_____

_____

d. Victim report of the accident, how the injury occurred, how she feels now and any other information. _____

_____

_____

10. This victim fell while skiing, extended her left arm to break the fall and dislocated her thumb. The thumb is pointed toward the wrist.

   a. Injury type(s) and location(s) _____

_____

_____

   b. Immediate first aid rendered _____

_____

_____

   c. Other information needed by medical professionals _____

_____

_____

   d. Victim report of the accident, how the injury occurred, how she feels now and any other information. _____

_____

_____

11. Caught in a slammed car door, this victim has a crush injury to fingers 3, 4 and 5 of his left hand. Each of the injured fingers is bent in the opposite direction at the second joint of the phalanges. There are several lacerations as well. The fingers are beginning to throb and the victim is in great pain.

   a. Injury type(s) and location(s) _____

_____

_____

   b. Immediate first aid rendered _____

_____

_____

   c. Other information needed by medical professionals _____

_____

_____

   d. Victim report of the accident, how the injury occurred, how she feels now and any other information. _____

_____

_____

12. This victim has hit her thumb with a hammer. The result is a growing hematoma under the thumbnail. The victim is in great pain and medical attention is not readily available.

a. Injury type(s) and location(s) _____

_____

_____

b. Immediate first aid rendered _____

_____

_____

c. Other information needed by medical professionals _____

_____

_____

d. Victim report of the accident, how the injury occurred, how she feels now and any other information. _____

_____

_____

13. This victim is an elderly man who has paralysis of his left side. His face is asymmetrical and his pupils are unequal in size.

a. Injury type(s) and location(s) _____

_____

_____

b. Immediate first aid rendered _____

_____

_____

c. Other information needed by medical professionals _____

_____

_____

d. Victim report of the accident, how the injury occurred, how she feels now and any other information. _____

_____

_____

14. This seventeen-year-old boy has been growing progressively sicker throughout the night. He has been complaining of abdominal pain. His discomfort has progressed to the point that he cannot find a comfortable position for rest or sleep. Your examination shows that he is hot to the touch, has taut abdominal muscles and is guarding his abdomen because even the slightest touch is painful.

a. Injury type(s) and location(s) _____

_____

_____

b. Immediate first aid rendered _____

_____

_____

c. Other information needed by medical professionals _____

_____

_____

d. Victim report of the accident, how the injury occurred, how she feels now and any other information. _____

_____

_____

15. You have administered CPR to an elderly woman. She now has a pulse and is breathing. She is semiconscious. What should the emergency caregiver do now?

a. Injury type(s) and location(s) _____

_____

_____

b. Immediate first aid rendered _____

_____

_____

c. Other information needed by medical professionals _____

_____

_____

d. Victim report of the accident, how the injury occurred, how she feels now and any other information. _____

_____

_____

16. This victim fell from construction scaffolding. He complains of pain in his lower back and shortness of breath. He has tingling in his legs and feet.

    a. Injury type(s) and location(s)   _____

_____

_____

    b. Immediate first aid rendered   _____

_____

_____

    c. Other information needed by medical professionals   _____

_____

_____

    d. Victim report of the accident, how the injury occurred, how she feels now and any other information.   _____

_____

_____

17. This elderly man fell in his home. He has apparently been trying to get help for some time. You find him on the kitchen floor, weak, disoriented and able to speak only haltingly. You notice that his right foot is turned at an unnatural angle.

    a. Injury type(s) and location(s)   _____

_____

_____

    b. Immediate first aid rendered   _____

_____

_____

    c. Other information needed by medical professionals   _____

_____

_____

    d. Victim report of the accident, how the injury occurred, how she feels now and any other information.   _____

_____

_____

18. This victim has run into and broken a newly-cleaned, sliding glass door. There is severe bleeding from a wound on the rear of her right leg just behind the kneecap. She says that there might be glass in the wound.

a. Injury type(s) and location(s) _____

_____

_____

b. Immediate first aid rendered _____

_____

_____

c. Other information needed by medical professionals _____

_____

_____

d. Victim report of the accident, how the injury occurred, how she feels now and any other information. _____

_____

_____

19. After hitting the underside of the dash in an auto accident, this victim complains of pain in his knee. He was on the passenger side of the car and was not wearing his seat belt. On gentle palpation, it feels as if his kneecap is broken in half.

a. Injury type(s) and location(s) _____

_____

_____

b. Immediate first aid rendered _____

_____

_____

c. Other information needed by medical professionals _____

_____

_____

d. Victim report of the accident, how the injury occurred, how she feels now and any other information. _____

_____

_____

20. This victim heard a snapping sound and felt his knee give as he rounded second base during a softball game. As you approach, he is holding his knee. He does not want you to move it at all.

a. Injury type(s) and location(s) _____

_____

_____

b. Immediate first aid rendered _____

_____

_____

c. Other information needed by medical professionals _____

_____

_____

d. Victim report of the accident, how the injury occurred, how she feels now and any other information. _____

_____

_____

21. Stepping off the curb during an evening walk around the block, this forty-year-old woman suffered a sprained ankle. The ankle has begun to swell, and bruises are beginning to develop as well. She cannot bear any weight on the injured ankle.

a. Injury type(s) and location(s) _____

_____

_____

b. Immediate first aid rendered _____

_____

_____

c. Other information needed by medical professionals _____

_____

_____

d. Victim report of the accident, how the injury occurred, how she feels now and any other information. _____

_____

_____

22. An industrial accident has crushed this worker's foot. The victim heard snapping as the foot was injured, and tissues are split and swollen.

a. Injury type(s) and location(s) _____

_____

_____

b. Immediate first aid rendered _____

_____

_____

c. Other information needed by medical professionals _____

_____

_____

d. Victim report of the accident, how the injury occurred, how she feels now and any other information. _____

_____

_____

23. This victim was hit by a car and has an open fracture of the right femur. There is profuse bleeding, and the injured leg is now several inches shorter than the victim's other leg.

a. Injury type(s) and location(s) _____

_____

_____

b. Immediate first aid rendered _____

_____

_____

c. Other information needed by medical professionals _____

_____

_____

d. Victim report of the accident, how the injury occurred, how she feels now and any other information. _____

_____

_____

24. Two linemen for the local power company have been the victims of electric shock. They were on ladders when the incident occurred. Victim One is touching the wire and appears to be in cardiac arrest. He has a serious burn on the hand that is touching the wire. The electricity may still be on. The other lineman, Victim Two, has burns on his arms. He is conscious but very disoriented.

For Victim One:

a. Injury type(s) and location(s) _____

_____

_____

b. Immediate first aid rendered _____

_____

_____

c. Other information needed by medical professionals _____

_____

_____

d. Victim report of the accident, how the injury occurred, how she feels now and any other information. _____

_____

_____

For Victim Two:

a. Injury type(s) and location(s) _____

_____

_____

b. Immediate first aid rendered _____

_____

_____

c. Other information needed by medical professionals _____

_____

_____

d. Victim report of the accident, how the injury occurred, how she feels now and any other information. _____

_____

_____

25. Three people have been injured in a car crash. Victim One is found on his back on the road near the car. He has a piercing injury to the chest, possibly from glass, and has bright red blood in his throat. Victim Two is in the back seat of the car. She is unconscious with shallow breathing and a weak pulse. Blood and clear fluid are present in her ears and nose. Victim Three was apparently the driver. His left lower leg has an open fracture, is bent at approximately a 30-degree angle and is bleeding severely.

The first task to be accomplished is to decide which victim should be attended first. Assuming that there are two rescuers, decide on the order in which the victims should be given first aid and for what types of injuries.

_____

_____

_____

_____

_____

_____

When the decision about order of giving first aid is made, describe the injury type(s) and location(s) correctly, describe the first aid provided and summarize any information needed by professional rescuers. Complete the following for each victim.

For Victim One:

a. Injury type(s) and location(s) _____

_____

_____

b. Immediate first aid rendered _____

_____

_____

c. Other information needed by medical professionals _____

_____

_____

For Victim Two:

a. Injury type(s) and location(s) _____

_____

_____

b. Immediate first aid rendered _____

_____

_____

c. Other information needed by medical professionals _____

_____

_____

d. Victim report of the accident, how the injury occurred, how she feels now and any other information. _____

_____

_____

For Victim Three:

a. Injury type(s) and location(s) _____

_____

_____

b. Immediate first aid rendered _____

_____

_____

c. Other information needed by medical professionals _____

_____

_____

d. Reports of the mechanisms of injury from victims (put the description together to arrive at the best summary).

_____

_____

_____

_____

_____

_____

_____

_____

GLOSSARY

ABC Assessment — Airway, Breathing and Circulation assessment make up the primary survey.

Abdominal Quadrants — This is the imaginary division of the abdomen into four equal parts. The division is made by drawing two imaginary lines, one horizontal and one vertical each of which divides the abdomen into two equal parts. The four segments are called the right upper quadrant, the left upper quadrant, the right lower quadrant, and the left lower quadrant. Remember the idea of right and left is from the patient's point of view.

Abrasions — An injury to the outer layer(s) of the skin caused by scraping. Abrasions are subject to infection but are otherwise not life threatening.

Activated Charcoal — A harmless substance that is used in the management of poisonings and overdoses to absorb a substance in order to prevent it from leaving the digestive tract, and to allow it to pass from the body.

Adipose — Fatty tissue used to store energy in the body. Also known as *fat*.

Afterbirth — Delivered from the uterus after the birth of a fetus, this is made up of the placenta, chorion and amnion, along with some blood and blood clots.

AIDS — Acquired Immune Deficiency Syndrome is a condition in which the immune system of the body loses function. AIDS is a sexually transmitted disease.

Air Embolism — The presence of air in a blood vessel which results in a blockage of flow. This is usually due to opening a vessel above the heart or accidently through intravenous injection with a hypodermic needle.

Amniotic Sac — A thin walled bag which holds fluid and the fetus during pregnancy. It is attached to the uterus and placenta.

Anaerobic — In the absence of air or oxygen. Certain types of pathogens require an anaerobic environment for growth.

Anaphylactic Shock — A form of shock seen when the body reacts to invasion by a foreign substance with an exaggerated response; systems commonly involved are the respiratory and central nervous.

Anatomical Obstruction — A blocking of the airway by a body part, usually the tongue.

Angulated fractures — An angulated fracture is a break where the extremity turns or bends away from its normal position.

Anxiety — A feeling of apprehension and fear.

Apnea — Not breathing.

Arterial Bleeding — Pulsing, bright red blood escaping from an injured artery.

Articulation — Refers to the coming together of two bone ends to form a joint.

Aspirate — The act of inhaling. In emergency settings usually associated with the inhalation of fluids into the lungs.

Auricle — The outer appendage of the ear.

Avulsions — A forceful tearing away of a body part.

Bandage — A means of securing a dressing on a wound site. A bandage may also provide pressure to aid in hemorrhage control.

Basal Skull Fracture — A break in the floor of the cranium which houses the brain. Indicated by the presence of raccoon and Battle's signs.

Battle's Signs — Bruising behind and below the ears, indicating a skull fracture.

Belly Breathing — Breathing which is not assisted by the diaphragm. This is usually noticed when the abdomen rises during respiration, but the chest does not.

Bilateral Movement — Movement (usually synchronized) occurring on both sides of the body.

Biological Death — The total absence of a heartbeat.

Bleeding — Escape of blood from the body.

Bloody Show — When the mucous plug that blocks the cervix during pregnancy is lost there is a loss of blood—tinged mucous. Many times this indicates the beginning of labor.

Blunt Trauma — Injury caused by collision of a body part with a solid object.

Braxton—Hicks Contractions — Also known as "false labor". These contractions begin early in pregnancy and stretch and prepare the uterus for delivery. The contractions get stronger and last longer as pregnancy progresses.

Burn — Injury to tissue caused by excessive heat or exposure to caustic chemicals.

Cafe coronary — Induced by choking on food. The lack of oxygen resulting from airway obstruction leads to cardiac arrest.

Capillary bleeding — bleeding from the small vessels that carry blood to all parts of the body and skin.

Cardiac arrest — Stoppage of the heart.

Cardiac Insufficiency — A situation in which the heart cannot pump enough blood to meet the body's needs.

Cardiogenic Shock — Shock resulting from the sudden reduction in output from the heart.

Carotid Artery — A major vessel supplying blood to the head. This artery can be felt in the neck.

Caustic — Something which burns, or eats away things by chemical action.

Cerebral Vascular Accident— CVA, a stroke.

Cerebrospinal — Referring to the brain or spinal cord.

Cervical Spine — Vertebrae of the neck.

Cervix — The portion of the uterus which protrudes into the vagina.

Clammy — Skin that feels clammy is cool, moist and sticky.

Closed wound — Injury to tissue resulting in bleeding inside the body (bruising)

Clotting Mechanism — The process of changing calcium, platelets and other factors in the blood into thrombin which eventually meshes with fiber in forming a semi-solid gel or clot.

Constricted — Made smaller.

Coagulated — The transformation of a liquid into a semi-solid gel.

Coma position — Fetal position.

Core — The vital organs of the body in the head and throat.

Corrosive — Something which dissolves or corrodes things by chemical action, especially used with metals.

Crepitus — Sensation of contact between bone ends.

Crowning — Bulging of the vagina just prior to presentation of the fetus at birth.

Cyanosis — Bluish coloration of the skin due to lack of oxygen.

Deacceleration injuries — Injuries caused by rapid stopping, as in car accidents.

Degree — Measurement of severity in burns.

Deoxygenated — Interruption of normal oxygen supply.

Diaphragm — A structure defining the bottom of the chest. The diaphragm is one of the key structures in breathing.

Dilated — Opened as wide as possible.

Dilation and Curettage — Dilation (opening) of the cervix and scraping of the lining of the uterus with a tool known as a curet, done to diagnose disease or remove fragments of the placenta which may remain attached after birth.

Dislocation — Removal of bones from their normal positions as defined by joints.

Dressing — A clean or sterile covering for a wound which is applied directly to the site of injury. The purpose of dressing is to protect the wound, stop bleeding, and prevent further contamination of the wound site.

Ectoderm — The outermost layer of cells in the developing fetus which eventually become the nervous system and special sensory organs.

Embolism — An occlusion of an artery. An air embolism would be the result of an air bubble forming in a vein, usually above the heart.

Emergency Care — Care given to the ill or injured enabling them to survive until medical care is available.

Emergency Medical Systems — Organized civil authorities providing emergency care.

Emetic — A substance which acts upon the central nervous system to stimulate the vomiting reflex.

Endoderm — The innermost layer of developing fetal cells from which some many internal organs and the linings of the trachea, lungs and gastrointestinal—intestinal tract are formed.

Envenomation — The injection of venom through the skin by an insect.

Epiglottis — A structure in the throat that covers the passage to the larnyx.

Epistaxis — Bleeding from the nose.

Extruded — Forced out.

Exudate — A clear liquid found underneath blisters.

Flail chest — Abnormal movement of the chest as a result of fractures to three or more ribs, each in more than one place is known as flail chest.

Fracture — A crack or break in a bone.

Frostbite — The damaging effect of extreme cold on body tissue, especially the skin and subcutaneous tissue. The effects are especially noticeable in exposed areas of poor circulation such as the ears, nose, fingers and toes.

Frothy — When air is introduced into a fluid, the fluid begins to bubble. Frothing of blood often occurs in blood associated with respiratory trauma.

Gag Reflex — An involuntary reaction to being touched in the posterior pharynx or soft palate. The reflex is much like the muscular action of vomiting.

Gastric Distention — The filling of the stomach with air. This usually occurs when artificial respiration is given for an extended period of time or when excessive pressure is used during ventilatory attempts.

Geometric Decrease — Getting less and less at an extremely rapid rate. Arithmetic decrease = 100, 99, 98; geometric = 100, 50, 25.

Gangrene — The death of tissue usually as the result of insufficient blood supply.

"Good Samaritan" Law — Statutes protecting one from liability when rendering emergency care in the proper manner.

Hallucinogenic — Any substance which causes changes in the brain chemistry resulting in perception of sights or sounds not actually present.

Head-to-Toe Assessment — Thorough, systematic examination of the body carried out to determine injuries.

Heat Exhaustion — Collapse, profuse sweating, often with nausea, resulting from a lack of water in hot weather.

Heat Stroke — A dangerous condition caused by the failure of the temperature-regulating mechanism of the body.

Hemorrhage — Severe bleeding.

Hyperglycemia — Too much glucose in the bloodstream, this condition is usually the result of too little insulin.

Hyperventilate — To breathe very rapidly and deeply for a prolonged period of time.

Hyphema — Hemorrhage into the anterior chamber of the eye.

Hypoglycemia — Too little glucose in the bloodstream, this is usually a result of an excessive amount of insulin.

Hypotension — Low blood pressure which results when the amount of blood in the circulating system is reduced by a significant amount.

Hypothermia — Reduction of core body temperatures to dangerously low levels as a result of prolonged exposure to cold temperatures.

Hypovolemic Shock — Shock due to a reduced amount of blood circulating in the body.

Hypoxia — Insufficient oxygen in the blood resulting in cyanosis, tachycardia, and confusion.

Impinging — Something impinges if it strikes or encroaches on something else.

Incised wound — A wound with smooth, precise edges, such as an incision a surgeon would make.

Ischiopubic bones — This is the joining of the bones of the ischium and the pubis of the pelvis. It is an articulation of the pelvic ring.

Laryngectomee — A person with an artificial airway surgically implanted at the base of the neck.

Lavage — To flush out an organ.

Lacerated wound — A jagged edged break in the skin.

Ligaments — Tissues that connect bone to bone.

Lingual — Having to do with the tongue.

Meningeal layers —The brain and spinal cord is contained within three layers of tissue: the dura, the mater, the arachnoid and the pia mater. The outer layer is the dura mater which is a tough inelastic layer that adheres to the skull. The middle layer is the arachnoid; this layer is separated from the dura mater by fluid. The arachnoid is thinner than the dura mater. The innermost layer is the pia cord and is richly supplied with blood vessels. The arachnoid and the pia mater are most susceptible to infection and irritation.

Meningitis — Infection or irritation of one of the meningeal layers.

Mesoderm — The middle layer of developing fetal cells which becomes bone, muscle and blood.

Nasopharynx: The part of the pharynx above the soft palate extending to the nasal opening to the pharynx.

Neurovascular — Having to do with the nerves and/or vessels.

Occlude — To close off or block is the act of occlusion.

Open wound — Any wound that includes a break in the skin.

Ophthalmologist — A medical doctor who specializes in treatment of the eye.

Overdose — Introduction of any substance with the intent of harm.

Palatal — Pertaining to the roof of the mouth.

Palpation — To gently examine by feeling with the fingertips.

Paradoxical breathing — Paradoxical breathing occurs when part or all of the lung moves in the opposite direction of what is normal. This movement compromises respiratory effectiveness, which if uncorrected, may lead to cardiovascular complications and/or death.

Paraplegia — Paralysis of the lower limbs.

Pedis — Pertaining to the foot.

Perfusion — An organ is said to be perfused with blood if a sufficient blood supply enters and supplies the organ, then leaves that organ carrying off wastes.

Peripheral Pulses — Pulses which are outside the central regions of the body.

Poisoning — Accidental introduction of a foreign substance into the body. There are four common routes: inhaled, ingested, contact with the skin or injection through the skin.

Position of function —To assume a normal non-postured position which allows for relaxation of a particular body part.

Posterior Pharynx — The back of the pharynx.

Pressure point — Areas on the body upon which pressure exerted from the outside can pinch off an artery against the bone.

Presenting Part — The part of the fetus which appears at the opening of the vagina at delivery.

Prosthesis — Something artificial made to replace a missing biological part.

Psychogenic shock — Shock due to emotional upset.

Puncture wounds — Wounds caused by small instruments such as nails or needles. Puncture wounds are highly susceptible to infection.

Quadraplegia — Paralysis of arms and legs.

Raccoon Signs — Bruises surrounding the eyes that look much like the mask of a raccoon.

Radius — The bone or artery on the thumb side of the forearm.

Regurgitate — To vomit or throw-up.

Respirations — The process of exchanging oxygen and carbon dioxide within the body's tissues.

Respiratory Distress — Difficulty in breathing.

Rule of Nines — A system for estimating the damage to surface tissue from burns.

Septic shock — Shock due to infection.

Septic — The presence of microorganisms in the blood. This is especially applied when the organisms have a poisonous effect when they die and decay.

Shell — Arms, legs, skin and muscles of the body . (See core.)

Shock Lung — Shortness of breath, rapid breathing and decreased oxygenation of arterial blood supplies, the end result of which is great damage to the lungs and possible death. May be the result of trauma, disease or shock.

Semi-Recumbent — Partially sitting up.

Septum — A partition or division, usually dividing a structure into halves.

Shock Lung — Shortness of breath, rapid breathing and decreased oxygenation of arterial blood supplies, the end result of which is great damage to the lungs and possible death. May be the result of trauma, disease or shock.

Spontaneous pneumothorax — Normally the result of chronic lung disease, spontaneous pneumothorax is a rupture of a weak spot on the lung.

Sprain — Damage to a joint.

Stoma — An opening in the body which has been surgically created. Examples would be the opening made in the trachea of a laryngectomee for breathing or the opening made in the abdominal wall for drainage in colostomy patients.

Strain — Damage to a muscle and/or tendon.

Syrup of Ipecac — A substance used in the management of poisonings and overdoses that acts on the chemical receptors of the brain in the medulla to produce vomiting.

Tendons — Tissues that connect muscle to bone.

Third Space — Extracellular fluid that is lost in a portion of the body where it cannot be used to fill the needs of the body.

Tourniquet — A rarely used hemorrhage control in which all circulation of blood to the injury is blocked.

Transportation Emergency: An injury which the rescuer can do nothing about, and which may deteriorate into a life-threatening emergency. These situations call for stabilization of the patient and immediate transport.

Triage — The process of deciding which victims need treatment first based on the severity of the injury and likelihood of recovery.

Trimesters — Pregnancy is divided into three periods of approximately three months each; each of the divisions is known as a trimester.

Umbilicus: The navel or belly button.

Vasoconstriction — Anything which causes the vessels diameter to decrease. This may be the result of drug ingestion, damage to the central nervous system, or the release of hormones within the body.

Vasodilation — Anything which causes the diameter of the vessels to increase. This may be the result of pooling of fluids in the vessels, the reaction to the body's own chemicals or hormones, or damage to the central nervous system.

Venous Bleeding — Bleeding from veins. This blood is usually dark red.

Ventilation — The process of moving gases into and out of the lungs.

Ventricles — The major pumping chambers of the heart or a cavity in the brain.

Vernix Caseosa — The wax—like covering of a fetus which protects it from the mineral content of amniotic fluids while it is in the uterus.

Vital Signs — Essential signs of life and health: pulse, respiration, blood pressure and temperature.

Vitreous Humour — The transparent jelly-like liquid which fills the posterior chamber of the eye.

Xiphoid Process — The pointed cartilaginous termination of the sternum.

INDEX

215